THE
YOGA
OF
WORKS

*Based on Sri Aurobindo's
Synthesis of Yoga*

TALKS AT CENTRE

1

M. P. PANDIT

Publisher:
LOTUS LIGHT PUBLICATIONS
P.O. BOX 2, WILMOT, WI 53192

First U. S. edition April 24, 1985

Published by Lotus Light by arrangement with Sri
M.P. Pandit

Cover Design: Dale Kappy

ISBN: 0-941524-21-3

Library of Congress Catalog Card Number: 85-50695

Printed in the United States of America

CONTENTS

PREFACE

This series of talks based on *The Synthesis of Yoga* of Sri Aurobindo was given at the Centre, Peace, Auroville from March 1972 to December 1973. The edited transcriptions of these meetings published here comprise the first of three volumes to be issued, corresponding to the four parts of *The Synthesis of Yoga:* " The Yoga of Divine Works "; " The Yoga of Integral Knowledge" and "The Yoga of Divine Love "; and " The Yoga of Self-Perfection ". The talks follow the sequence of the original work, though there are seventeen of them here for the thirteen chapters; several of the chapter titles in this work are the same as those in *The Synthesis of Yoga.* Most of the presentations are followed by questions and answers covering a wide range of spiritual topics not necessarily directly related to the theme of the talks.

1

THE FOUR AIDS

I am sure many of you have heard of the great epic of India called the Mahabharata. It concerns the legendary fight between the hosts of light, justice and truth, and the hosts of darkness, injustice and falsehood. These powers striving for supremacy are embodied in the two hosts of princes, the Kurus and the Pandavas. Destiny lies symbolically in the hands of an emperor who is blind. During the course of the pourparlers before the war breaks out, there is an emissary from the camp of the Pandavas to the emperor. The king has taken an obviously untenable position and the emissary tells him point blank, at the late hour of the night when he has arrived, that what he has to say will be told in public the next day. The king is perturbed, calls his counsellor and asks him to say some soothing words. The minister—Vidura is his name—embodied Knowledge. He tells the king that no words the human mouth could utter would soothe him, but to answer his questions, to meet his difficulties, he will summon a divine sage, Sanatsujata. The minister concentrates in yoga and invokes the presence of the sage. And the first question that the king asks is, "Is there death, or death is not?"

The answer of Rishi Sanatsujata is, "Death is and death is not."

"And what is death?"

"Death" he declares, "is heedlessness. Inattention, not to be aware, that is death. When you are not aware, when you are not heedful, you fall from your true nature—that is death. When you are aware you rise above death."

"How to be aware? Of what to be aware?"

"Be aware of your divine nature, of the divine truth behind all things."

"How is that knowledge to be attained? How is one to remember and realise one's own true nature, true reality?"

The sage replies, "There are four indispensable aids: *knowledge* of what you want to realise; the *teacher* who is to communicate the knowledge; zeal and *practice*, the personal effort to realise the knowledge that has been communicated; and *time*, the instrumentality of time. These are the four essential ingredients of the spiritual adventure."

Sri Aurobindo recalls this passage in his small but significant book, *The Yoga and Its Objects*. He recalls the same truth in the first chapter of *The Synthesis of Yoga* which he has entitled, "The Four Aids". As you are aware, the series on *The Synthesis of Yoga* appeared simultaneously with that on *The Life Divine* in the pages of the "Arya" nearly sixty years ago. He gave in *The Life Divine* the metaphysics, the knowledge of the gospel of divine life. But he was not content with giving the knowledge, he accompanied it with a series, *The Synthesis of Yoga,* illustrating the method of translating this knowledge into practice. Unless knowledge in the mind is translated in practical terms, made real to the rest of the being, it remains a theory, a book-knowledge with no effective consequence in life.

The first essential in the situation is *knowledge*. Knowledge of what? And what is knowledge? Science.

literature, humanities, are they the knowledge that is spoken of here? In one of the old Upanishads there is a legend that sage Narada, the Divine Singer, realises at one time that all his proficiencies in the various sixty-four branches of systematised knowledge are not adequate. He prays and invokes the sage of whom we just spoke, Sanatsujata, and tells him, "I have read, I have studied, I have acquired proficiency in all these sixty-four branches of learning," he narrates them one by one and continues, "but still I do not know; would you give me the knowledge by which I may know?" And the story goes that the divine sage revealed to him the knowledge of the essential principles of existence, the knowledge by which all other knowledge becomes real.

In another Upanishad there is a clear distinction made between the lower knowledge and the higher knowledge. The lower knowledge includes the field covered by most of our sciences and arts; it relates not to the fundamentals but to the processes. All our sciences, all our arts relate to the process, to the way in which things take shape, move, develop. But what the things *are* is not considered. The Upanishad declares that the knowledge which gives you, which enables you to know, the fundamental reality of things, the basis of things by knowing which all is known—*yasmin vijnate sarvam idam vijnatam*—that is *para vidya,* that is the higher knowledge.

So the real knowledge relates to the soul of things, to the basic reality. And that knowledge is not to be gained from books. It is a knowledge that reveals itself to the prepared and equipped mind. One cannot seize or grasp it, one cannot make inroads by one's intellect. But to one who is purified and silent, that knowledge reveals itself, unveils itself.

There have been great men, great mystics, who
have been vouchsafed such high knowledge at different
times and occasions in the history of humanity. And
part of the knowledge that they have thus received
they have formulated in terms of the intellect so that
the human mind could understand something of it,
could find through this a bridgehead to the deeper
knowledge. This formulation of the supreme transcendent knowledge in terms of the human intellect, in
human language, is called in India the *shastra*—the
scripture, the authentic word.

A seeker of the divine path, such as the Integral
Yoga with which we are concerned in our study, has first
to know something of this knowledge. What is the
knowledge that supports and bases this line of yoga?
Is it one textbook, one scripture like the Veda, the Gita
or the Bible? There are so many, and indeed each one
contains a particular presentation of the higher truth
suited to the mentality of the age and section of humanity to which it was addressed. The seeker of the
Integral Yoga does not confine himself to one scripture,
to one text. He sees, he studies this knowledge of the
reality—of God, of Nature, of himself—wherever it is
found, wherever it appeals to him. He delves into it,
familiarises himself with the main concepts and fundamentals. This is one aspect from the human approach.

A deeper aspect of the situation is that all this knowledge that can be gathered through books is partial, it
does not exhaust the whole of knowledge. There is within
each one a seed of knowledge. There is embedded in
man a spark of divinity. Along with the spark there is
also the seed of knowledge of that divinity. It is the
function of the shastra to awaken the heart and direct
the mind of the individual to that centre of knowledge

within him lying veiled behind curtains and curtains of ignorance. The individual has to purify himself, to concentrate, to invoke the inner knowledge to reveal itself. All his understanding, all his study of the written word is a preparation. The spoken word is a door opening on the word unspoken. Only a small fraction of the totality of knowledge finds expression in verbal terms.

This done, an initial entry made into the realms of knowledge, the next step is to find a *teacher*. In all spiritual traditions the teacher, the *guru* as we call him in India, occupies a pivotal place. The teacher in the spiritual quest is not an instructor. He is not a director who tells you what to do, who shows you the way to libraries and books, and whose duty to you is done once you are out of the classroom. A teacher is regarded in the Indian tradition as someone even more than a father. It is declared in the Tantric scriptures that parents give you a human birth but the teacher gives you a birth into the spirit of God. His is a greater service than that of the father. And a guru represents to the disciple, to the seeker, the very godhead, the very divinity to which he aspires. Whatever may be the perfections or the imperfections of the teacher from the human level, the disciple opens to the divine part in the teacher when he accepts him as a guru. He is not merely fascinated by, attracted or bound to, the human side, it is something divine in the teacher, something with which the soul of the disciple has affinity, that attracts him. The true link is between the divine part of the teacher and the soul of the disciple. Through this central part the divine knowledge, the divine reality to which one aspires, emanates; it pours upon the disciple. When the teacher is satisfied that a seeker is intended to be his disciple and that he is intended by the Divine to be its channel to reach him, he decides in which line of yoga, in which line of spiritual effort the novice is to be initiated. He observes the seeker—his nature, his stage of evolutionary development, his aspiration, the direction of his soul—and chooses the precise line into which he is to be initiated.

This initiation is a highly fascinating subject. There are as many as sixteen modes of initiation. It is not necessary for our purpose to go into too much detail about these diverse modes. All that should be understood is that there is not one way of initiation. The traditional way familiarised in India of the teacher whispering some *mantra* or word into the ear of the disciple is only one way. There are many others. The teacher just thinks of the disciple and an impact is made; something of the spiritual dynamism of the teacher impinges upon him and sets going a spiritual motor in his heart. Or he looks and in the very sight a contact is made. Or he touches the disciple—there is a physical transmission. And so on, there are various methods which are open to the spiritual teacher.

People ask me in person or through correspondence: "How are we to be sure that the Mother has accepted us as her disciples? She has not given us a mantra, she has not touched us and said, 'You are initiated.'" I am obliged to tell them that hers is not the usual, traditional way, she has many ways of initiating, of accepting the seeker as a disciple. But one thing she has said is that when you accept her as your teacher, you may take it that you are automatically accepted by her as her disciple. The onus is upon the seeker; the sincerity with which he accepts her decides the depth upon which his discipleship stands.

By whatever means the teacher accepts the seeker as his disciple, it is graphically described in the mystic tradition of India that the teacher takes him into his own being. When the disciple is thus taken in, there is formed a foetus, as it were; he stays in the womb for a full three days (three is a significant figure) and thereafter when the spiritual child is born the very gods are present to greet the newcomer. The past human birth and life is left behind and he is born into a new life. This is the role of the teacher—to give a new birth to the disciple. All knowledge that you get by reading, that you have acquired by your own effort—the book knowledge, the mental knowledge—is energised by the touch of the teacher. What is confusing or not relevant gets cleared, gets eliminated, and the knowledge that is already present acquires a full light. And from the being of the teacher there is a continuous charge of illumination to different points of the disciple's being pouring flames of knowledge. The teacher, Sri Aurobindo describes, does not arrogate to himself a superior position demanding obedience from the disciple. An ideal teacher is one who does not dictate. There is his teaching, there is his example; he is there embodying the ideal which you seek to realise. That he is present in concrete form is itself a great encouragement, a standing power to inspire the disciple. There is, besides, his continuous influence, known and unknown to the disciple. There is an incessant radiation of the spiritual vibrations of the teacher falling upon all in his surroundings, creating an effortless atmosphere of progress, of growth towards the ideal.

There is the knowledge; there is the teacher; third, it will not do only to read and stay in the presence of the guru, one has to make an *effort*. There is a controversy

among the learned people as to what is the role of personal effort, and what the role of grace. Is it grace that
achieves or is it effort? Is it not true that the ultimate
sanction has to come from above, is it not true that you
can't storm the gates of heaven by your zeal? After all,
is not human zeal an effervescence? That is one standpoint. The other is: the grace is always there, the grace
is pouring but there must be somebody, there must be
something done at our level, to receive the grace. There
is a downpour of rain but the field has to be ready. It has
to be made ready: the ground has to be dug, the weeds
have to be removed, the seed must be there. So, from
the human side preparation is indispensable. This controversy is never solved satisfactorily at the academic level
because the mistake is made of looking upon effort and
grace as two contradictory, two unconnected, truths.
When once, long ago, the Mother was asked what answer
she had to give to this question, she said grace and effort
are two ends of the same truth: because there is grace
one is impelled to do the effort. One is moved to think
of higher things, one is inspired to strive for higher things
because there is an impulsion from grace. And because
there is effort from here, the grace responds more and
more. They are interconnected. Mother once said (I do
not quote her exact words but what she said in substance)
that without effort things remain stagnant, without grace
things remain unfruitful; there is an interaction of effort
and grace. And what is the effort that man is called upon
to put in? It is the effort of aspiration—aspiration for
the higher truth; rejection—rejection of all that is contrary to that truth or stands in the way of realising that
truth; and surrender—surrender of oneself to the higher
truth embodied either in the teacher or felt on the heights
or in the depths of one's being, surrender to a divine

power whether in a human form or not. This triple labour of aspiration, rejection, and surrender constitutes the personal and human effort.

But human effort is not going to achieve things in a day, nor is the grace going to perform miracles every day. In fact there are no miracles. What appears as a miracle, you can be sure, is the fine result of a long long preparation that has gone on before—either in this birth or the previous birth or more. There is the instrumentality of *time*. We are in a universe governed by space and time. Time is a great determinant. There is an intelligence behind time, a consciousness; it knows the precise hour when you are ready for the realisation. One shall not complain of the time required to achieve a result for which evolutionary nature, unaided by human effort and divine grace, would take millions of years. Time shall not be stinted; one has to know how to wait. As the Mother has said somewhere, to know how to wait is to put time on your side; time is your friend, time is an obstruction, it all depends upon your attitude. If you function from the level of your ego—that you are doing everything, that by your effort, your knowledge, your dynamism, you are going to achieve—time comes in your way and forces you to test your claim at every step. Were you to surrender yourself to a higher force—to the divine *shakti*, to the divine puissance—forget yourself (or as they put it, "die to yourself"), detach yourself from the ego and let yourself be carried as a surrendered child by the Divine Mother, time turns out to be a friend. Time, then, goes so quickly, it is so helpful; time is a hastener. The ideal attitude for the seeker—as Sri Aurobindo has declared more than once—is to have patience as if the whole of eternity is there before you, and yet at the same time to summon and develop all the energies

that you have with an intensity and rapidity as if you
have to achieve your goal the next moment.

Any questions?

Is it always necessary to have a physical guru?

I would answer that when it concerns a living teacher
or a teaching that is fresh—when the teacher is alive
physically or his influence and force are still dynamic
on Earth—one can always start by reading his books, by
reading his words. It is only if one does not correctly
understand the message or the directions in the book
that a physical guru is advisable. The books of Sri
Aurobindo and the Mother do not normally need the
intercession of a physical guru. They are so framed, the
knowledge is so layed out, that the influence of the
teacher is there in every word. It is going to be that way
for a long time. If you accept this book, *The Synthesis of
Yoga,* as your guide, you automatically accept Sri
Aurobindo as your teacher.

I have received a remarkable letter written by a
gentleman from the U.S.A. He has never been here. He
read some of the books of Sri Aurobindo—I think they
were the letters to disciples—and decided he should
practise this yoga. Things started happening which will
illustrate what power a living word has. This gentleman
has not read many of the books of Sri Aurobindo or the
Mother; I don't think he even knows of the existence of
the Mother. He seems to be a businessman. He read
these books, sat down and started concentrating on the
Divine as Love. He excluded every other idea from his
mind. For half an hour or so every day he would think of
the Divine as Love. Surprisingly, things began to happen.
From the centre of his heart there was a continuous

unrolling of waves of love. They embraced all around, the whole universe; they started going up. But this required certain application, concentration, and devotion of time which he could not spare. So he thought that was not his way. Then he thought the way of knowledge could be his. He read the relevant portions and started gathering his consciousness in the mind. Here too things started. He felt his consciousness separating itself from the mind, going up and up. He says there were pillars of light, things were pouring down. He felt a thrill, a continuous sense of delight. And when things were going in this way, he began to feel he was being inundated and *he* would be lost. He got afraid and stopped the experience. And he asked: "Am I doing the right thing? What am I to do if I die?"

It was a right movement. I am sorry the gentleman has mistaken things. He was on the verge of a capital experience when the fear came in. And this fear of death, of self-loss, is really the fear of the ego.

This experience has occurred many times here in the Ashram; Sri Aurobindo himself has spoken of it in his conversations. A gentleman came to him one day—long before Sri Aurobindo retired—and said, "I want to meditate but thoughts disturb me." Sri Aurobindo told him to sit down and close his eyes. Things started happening. The man's mind became blank, quiet, there was a rock of peace settling in, no movement. Suddenly the man shouted, "I am dying!" And Sri Aurobindo says he was not so patient in those days and he had to let the man lose that remarkable experience.

The American gentleman's experience shows that there is a dynamic power in these books which one can receive and follow. He had not read fully, that is why he let go of that experience. I have written to him explaining matters, that he should not be afraid, that he should let himself be carried by the Divine Force that is claiming him.

So it is not always necessary to accept a physical guru unless one feels one's limitations to grasp and follow the teaching.

In the section on time in the first chapter there is one sentence I found confusing. It says, "Time is a field of circumstances and forces meeting and working out a resultant progression whose course it measures." Would you please explain?

This earth which is the field of manifestation is thereby a field of the clash, friction, and working out of innumerable possibilities that have been released into action. There are a million possibilities in the bosom of the infinite. Some of them are released. They clash; each one tries to realise itself as if it alone exists. And out of this clash of possibilities, working together at certain junctures, the result emerges. That is why one can never predict on Earth what particular result will come to be at a particular time. The various possibilities of the working—possibilities that are not patent but latent—are always there. And time is the background across which all these possibilities are turning, revolving, clashing and working out some result. Circumstance is one part, one feature of this situation, one juncture in the realisation of certain possibilities. Between the struggle of possibilities and the realisation of an actuality there is time, there is a lapse of time. Time measures it. And all this work of the clash of possibilities is directed from within with a view to ensure the evolutionary progress of all that is involved in this manifestation. Evolution itself is a result of struggle. There are forces and possibilities that help, possibilities that oppose. There is always a friction. Human nature, being what it is, gives enough scope for this clash. Time is the measurer; time observes; time contains. There is no such clash and struggle on the higher planes. It is here in the field of evolution that the possibilities are deliberately released for working themselves into actualities. There are a million casualties; only a few possibilities succeed in realising themselves.

Could you say that these forces themselves as they interact are or create time?

No. The forces that interact are not all simple forces, many are presided over by certain beings from the subtler planes. They are anterior to time. Time and space of which he speaks here relate to the Earth-field. Other levels have their own time, their own space. But he is speaking only of the Earth-field, and these possibilities are anterior.

How is one to resolve the dilemma of thinking on one hand about transformation, about change, about the future, and on the other hand to live fully in the moment?

Man is not of one piece. Man lives simultaneously on different levels of his being. Day to day effort, living in the moment and the movement not concerned with the next moment, has to be on the dynamic and working level. But on the contemplative level, which can be simultaneously active, one has to create the mental atmosphere, the mental climate for transformation, for change—to think of what the change is going to be, of what it expects of one, what is likely to be demanded of one in the future. So in that way the mind has to be active in a progressive direction thus giving a constant lead to the practical part which is concerned with moment to moment effectuation of the ideal. One has to invoke, act, aspire, feel, plan and think, and one has to be absolutely detached and passive. All these have to be done simultaneously. Man is a multiple being and to be multiply functioning is his very nature.

What I find is that if I start thinking about transformation or the future, then those rare times of silence during which one really gets into the moment just dissolve. And suddenly you realise that you may be worrying about some change that is going to happen, or anticipating it or hoping for it, and then an anxiety gets created.

There is a question of striking a balance, keeping a balance between the different activities. Regarding the particular question that you pose: it is not really in human hands to effect the transformation. The transformation of human nature is to be achieved by a Force and a Power greater than the human. What is demanded of man is an utter, unquestioning receptivity. Our responsibility ceases the moment we are truly surrendered. It is not our problem whether the transformation is going to be today or tomorrow or not at all this time. It is in greater hands than ours. They know the time, they know the hour. We should not be found wanting when the moment comes. Our vision, our effort should be confined to keeping ourselves ready—to keep the mind clear, without confusion, to know exactly what transformation means and what it expects of us, and do it. To do anything beyond that is an indulgence in mental acrobatics.

There is a condition where someone has in the mind a sense of understanding of what should be done, and another in which one is actually in the condition of doing it. How can one know that it is not just in the mind alone that one is engaged, projecting that that fact is taking place when it may not really be?

It is a ticklish problem because a person who sees it in the mind, at the mental level, has the conviction that it is *the* way. But whether another mind may not see it in another way, and what is the right way, that has to be tested empirically. What the mind sees or feels need not be immediately true. The circumstances for its being realised may not be ready. So one has to wait, one has to watch, one has to compare and see if that sense of certitude which springs from the heart backs up the mental vision. A mental certainty won't do. If there is a conviction and a self-evident certitude that comes here [gesture pointing to the heart or psychic centre], and if you're sure this is *that* and nothing else, you can be convinced that what you are seeing is true and the right way for you.

But there are conditions when one can be out of synchronisation and imagines on the mental plane that the thing is really happening in the other areas of the being when it very well may not be. How to escape that?

I understand. There is what is called in yoga a purely mental formation. On that level it is true, you feel it to be true. But at the first touch of concrete reality outside it breaks down. All that is weaved, all that is concretely experienced in the mind need not be actual, it can be a mental fabrication or formation. This particularly happens with those who have an imaginative turn of mind or are given to certain grand eloquent dreams—the stress of ego. The mind weaves, it takes up certain ideas, desires, and makes patterns. All that can be said is that a robust common sense has to be the barometer in most mental experiences. A genuine spiritual experience does not need any barometer, it is self-evident. But a mental experience, however brilliant it may be, has to be

subjected to the canons of common sense and then only
verified and accepted.

When one discovers the inner certitude, the inner authority,
should one still obey any external authority such as books for
instance?

If one can be sure that it is not a mental formation
or an egoistic projection but is the voice of the inner,
true soul, that should be given precedence over the
written word. If you are fortunate to have a teacher, to
have a guru, such matters are to be referred to him and
the guidance sought. But the written word can never be
the final thing.

2

INITIATION AND SELF-CONSECRATION

This is Sri Aurobindo's epigram of the chapter: "He who chooses the Infinite has been chosen by the Infinite." This perception has a great bearing on the practical side of spiritual life. It means that one thinks of the Divine because the Divine has already thought of him. One thinks of God when one's evolutionary development has reached a stage when he can take the godward turn. Whatever may be the apparent reason that is responsible for one's turning to spiritual life, the fact remains that one thinks of the higher life because one is ready for it. An implication of this truth is that once you take sincerely to spiritual life of whatever pattern, you cannot with impunity go back from it. It is not like choosing a profession or selecting a subject for study and dropping it when you find it difficult or find something else more attractive or lucrative. Here it is a question of the soul. The soul has decided and it has pushed you into the spiritual life. If for any reason, due to weakness in any part of the being, you decide to go back to the ordinary life, it means you betray the soul. And under these circumstances the consequences are bound to be disastrous. If a person who has received the true call to the Divine turns his back after that, the soul exerts its pressure; there is a disharmony between the external being which has turned away and the soul which has chosen the path. This disharmony reflects itself either in the form of illness or depression, or it invites accidents or disasters.

Another point to be added is that everyone has the Guide within. There is the world-teacher stationed in the core of the heart of every individual, but one is not normally conscious of that presence. There are veils after veils of ignorance preventing a direct communion with the inner teacher. This being a common human frailty, Sri Aurobindo describes the helpful role that an external teacher plays in the spiritual life of the seeker.

The first type of this external aid, which alone is recognised by the physical eye accustomed to the concrete realities of matter, is the chosen *form* of God. Each one has a preference, a natural tendency or liking for one particular form among the many under which the Divine has been worshipped down the ages. It may be Christ, it may be Krishna, Shiva or Buddha, but whatever the form, there is a certain affinity between the soul that aspires and the God-form that is adored or worshipped.

For those who may not have this link of communion with the Divine in form, there is the *avatar*. An avatar is a manifestation of God for purposes of creation. In order to help the course of the spiritual evolution of the world, to negotiate certain crucial turns of the progression, the Divine takes human form and works out the difficulty. He establishes the fact of the conquest of that particular difficulty and gives a new turn to the course of the spiritual evolution of humanity. There have been a number of such avatars. A real avatar, a true manifestation—nowadays there are dozens of "avatars" in the world as you are all aware—is one who is conscious of his divinity from the very beginning of his life. He is not an evolving being who realises God. It is God himself who takes a poise and an embodiment suited to the particular stage of development of humanity, suited to the problems that are to be solved. Avatars are direct manifestations of the Divine who have played a crucial role in the development of humanity. A seeker may derive inspiration by worship and adoration of, by meditation on, these avatars or their teachings.

The third type of external teacher is the *prophet*. Prophets are world-teachers who do not claim to be avatars. They are not direct manifestations of the Divine. A prophet is a chosen vehicle for the communication of a divine wisdom, a divine power, to those who are ready for it. Moses and Mohammed are standing examples in history of world prophets.

Then comes the *guru*, the human teacher, the human representative of the Divine to the disciple. As I said last time, the guru is not an instructor, he is something more, even something more than a human father. In the Tantric tradition in India, there are interesting analyses of the various types of gurus. There is what is called the *siksa* guru, the guru who expounds and teaches the shastra to the enquiring intelligence and equips the mind with an ordered knowledge bearing on the meaning and goal of existence. He gives you the formulated knowledge in words. He sees what knowledge is suited to your frame of mind and he directs you to that. There is also the *diksa* guru, he who initiates the seeker into the dynamics of the path that is to be followed to translate that knowledge into his own life. A more detailed classification of the types of gurus specifies six different categories: the *preraka*, who creates an interest in sadhana, the practical discipline, by drawing attention to its beneficent results—he stimulates your interest in spiritual life and no more; the *sucaka*, who opens the eye of the seeker to the vision of the sadhana and its objective—it is one step more, beyond mere interest, he makes you see the truth of sadhana, the beauty of sadhana, the need for sadhana; the *vacaka*, who explains

the method and the goal; the *darsaka,* who shows these
details in a convincing manner, step by step; the *siksaka,*
who undertakes to teach the novice day by day; and
then, the *bodhaka,* who imbues the aspirant with the
necessary understanding of mind and illuminates his
being with his own spiritual light. These are the different
categories of gurus recognised in the Tantric tradition.
You would have seen that the born guru embodies the
capacities of all these six types in himself; depending
upon the stage at which the disciple has arrived, the
guru plays this role or that.

And the way the guru helps the disciple is through
diksa, initiation. Initiation may be external, *kriya diksa,*
effected through some outer means of interchange—
the giving of a book, a present, a flower—there is a ritual
conducted and through it the guru places himself in a
relation with the disciple. Or there is initiation through
an inner and subtle means, *abhyantari;* it is not seen,
there is no outer ceremony or exchange but there is an
inner impact, *vedha diksa*—the arrow falls on the target.
It is called *vedha* because like the hunter reaching his
prey by sheer sound-direction, without even seeing his
object, the guru's power strikes at the being of the disciple
wherever he is, irrespective of any barrier or distance.
Initiation without ritual is again threefold: *sparsi,*
based upon touch, tends the disciple in the manner
of a bird nourishing its young ones within the warm
folds of its wings—brooding over them, it brings them
to birth; *caksusi,* based upon sight, acts like the fish who
brings up its offspring by means of sight alone—there
is a belief that the mother fish raises its young by looking at them, that through the gaze it gives nourishment;
manasi, based upon the mind, builds like the tortoise
feeding its infants by only thinking of them—its young

ones are spread here and there, it is a slow moving creature so it sits in one place and thinks of them, and in the very process of thinking a subtle nourishment is reached to them. These are the three types of initiation which a guru can give—by touch, by sight, by thought.

There is yet another classification which categorises the initiation threefold. *Shakti* is that in which there is no ritual or physical contact for purposes of initiation. It takes place when the guru by his yogic power enters his own shakti, consciousness-force, into the being of the disciple directly. The disciple may not even be physically present before the guru. The guru thinks of him and sends an emanation of his consciousness to enter and take charge of the initiate. Another and more pregnant is *sambhavi*, the contact that takes place at the mere sight of the guru, by just a touch or an exchange of words, and brings about something like a revolution in the consciousness of the disciple precipitating the advent of a divine pervasion. The third is *mantri*, in which a mantra or ritual or any kind of perceptible means is used to forge the relation. A mantra is whispered in secrecy into the ear of the disciple. Along with the mantra, something of the consciousness of the initiator enters into the being of the disciple and keeps alive the mantra for the rest of his life.

Though not strictly relevant to our purpose, I thought you would be interested to know what the Indian tradition has to say on the subject.

These points included, we may now pass to the second chapter, " Self-Consecration ".

It is not difficult to enter the spiritual path by some means, to give up the ordinary life and take to the spiritual. The entry may be caused by some relation with, or admiration or fascination exercised by, a teacher or an advanced seeker. It may come by reading something that creates interest in the truth that is propounded, and one wishes to realise it. One may get a shock from a death or some disaster, it suddenly cuts the knot tying you to the lower life and you are freed. There are many other ways in which one may turn to spiritual life. It is a universal experience that when one does turn to yoga, to spiritual life of any kind, there is a sense of elation, there is a sense of newness, worthwhileness. And one feels inspired, open to waves of bliss, to the touch of peace, to the throb of power, and much more. But after this initial period of enthusiasm passes, there is an interregnum of depression, difficulty, troubles. That is because usually the decision to live a higher life is taken by only one part of the being: it may be the awakened mind, it may be the emotional heart which flows towards the teacher or the ideal embodied in the teacher, it may be just an idea that captures the imagination. But unless steps are taken to extend the area of this spiritual living, the other parts rise in revolt, they go on strike and insist on returning to their petty rounds. One has to take the trouble in the earlier stages to train the other parts of the being to collaborate with the central part that has chosen. One has to read favourable literature, accustom the mind to the higher vibrations and train the heart to expand itself, to extend its emotions and love, train the life-energies to dedicate themselves in the cause of the Divine, train the very body to look upon itself as a pedestal for the edifice of God under erection. Unless this step is taken to follow up the initial choice, things get bogged down. This process of working out in detail the decision to surrender to a higher power is called *consecration*. Consecration is a detailed working out of the will for surrender that has been effected in the central part of the being.

It happens that some find that the difficulties are insurmountable. Their lower nature is not ready. The inspiration that led them to the path turns out to be temporary. Or at any rate, they cannot negotiate the difficulty. It is here that the aid of the guru, the help of the Grace, comes in. But even if an individual cannot profit by the help and assistance offered to him due to his inherent weaknesses, there is no lasting loss. Every forward step that has been taken is a gain. In the Bhagavad Gita it is said that no holy act, no forward step ever goes to waste; one degree has been gained. If one cannot summon enough sincerity to follow the path, he begins in the next birth at the point where he now leaves off. One should not regret at any time that one has taken to the spiritual path but has not been able to pursue it.

Everything ultimately is not decided by one's imperfections or weaknesses but by one's sincerity. To the weakest among us—if we can submit sincerely the problems to the teacher, the guru, the Divine—there is a flooding of the necessary strength that enables us to get over the difficulty. The question is, are we sincere? Are we sincere in praying to God to help us to overcome the difficulty? And sincerity has been defined by the Mother as a unification of the whole being around one purpose, around the chosen ideal. Any default, any backsliding at any level, means insincerity.

It is because of the problems raised by elements involved in ordinary life, by the lower nature which refuses to cooperate or change, that in many of the ancient and past traditions renunciation was called for.

It was said that there is a permanent dichotomy between spiritual life and worldly life. One has to renounce the world and all that belongs to it if one wants to lead a life consecrated to the Divine. This was an easy enough process, but it has been disastrous in countries like India who have seriously followed it. It is not difficult to renounce material possessions, worldly interest, to turn one's back on what has been given by God, and seek to realise him in one's nakedness. Even renunciation, asceticism, has a peculiar joy of its own which forms the vanity that, "I have renounced, I am a superior being to all those around me who are still involved and lost in the pleasures and movements of life." The Mother once said that in her whole life she had not seen more egoistic beings than some sannyasins. I have met them at very close quarters; what vanity—a suicidal spiritual vanity—some of them have, it is to be seen to be believed.

Renunciation in any case is not the way of this path; we embrace the Divine integrally. Beauty, splendour, power, wealth, are all special emanations of the Divine. And if we choose an integral Divine for our realisation, it stands to reason that we recognise and perceive the Divine in all the elements that constitute worldly prosperity and material wealth—for even matter is the robe of the spirit. The world is a manifestation of God.

3

CONSECRATION

Yoga is not to be taken as a pastime or a technique to be developed in one's spare hours, it is a full-time occupation, indeed, a preoccupation. Yoga is a new birth, a birth out of the limited existence in ignorance and imperfection into the vaster life of light, knowledge and bliss.

The door of entry into yoga is not the same for everyone. It can come in many ways. One may awaken to the truth of yoga and the necessity of practising it as a result of some inner door opening, as a result of an impact from a mighty personality, or some blow in life forcing one to see the impermanence of worldly existence as it is. One awakens to the possibility of leading a larger and a deeper life not susceptible to the shock of circumstances in external life. Whatever the door of entry, it is imperative that the whole being must take to yoga. At any rate, the Integral Yoga demands that there has to be an integral acceptance. Yoga cannot be practised only in one part. The mind, the heart, the will, the body, all have to assent to the demands of yoga and collaborate with goodwill towards the cultivation of yogic values.

The first condition for doing yoga is to reverse the direction of our existence. Normally the eye of man, the mind of man, is turned externally, outward, extrovert. By persistent will our energies have to be turned internally, inward, they have to be introverted and directed towards the soul.

This yoga does not seek an individual salvation beyond the world in a paradise elsewhere, it does not reject life as a falsehood or as an inferior existence. It looks upon the world and the universe as a manifestation of God. The world has to be fully possessed— possessed in the spirit and light and consciousness of its maker. We recall Sri Aurobindo's exhortation: " Reject not the body of God, O God-lover, but keep it for thy joy; for His body too is delightful even as His spirit."

After accepting this broad perspective of our effort, we awake in the process of yoga, in the process of self-observation, self-purification, and self-discovery to see that we are not what we normally think ourselves to be. We are normally aware of only our surface personality. This personality is nothing but a conglomeration of various thoughts, emotions, feelings, and movements held together by the linchpin that is the shadowy figure of ego. When we look within ourselves at the outset of yoga, we become aware that we are not one but we are many. When we look inside we become aware that there is a mind which has an existence of its own, a heart which has its own emotions and does not consult or depend upon the mind, a vast life-energy which functions as it likes, a physical body which though distinct is tyrannised by both the mind and life. There are so many complex personalities within each of us. We have to observe and disengage each part from the others and treat it to the higher or inner light.

We also become aware that we are not alone. When we observe our thoughts we see that only a fraction of them have been born in ourselves. We are constantly open to waves after waves of thought invasions from the universal atmosphere. They come unknown, unobserved, and take shape in our thought substance giving us the illusion that we are thinking *our* thoughts, *our* feelings. Actually, if we were to look behind the veil of the physical body we would see how defenceless we are against the constant flux of the universal life, mind, and heart that pour through us, cross through us at various levels. The seeker begins to awake to the enormity of the problem, for here he has to control, he has to check, he has to answer not for his own thoughts and emotions alone, but he has to be aware and take cognisance of the constant invasion of fresh thoughts and feelings coming from outside. And man, being an evolutionary being, has to carry the burden of the Earth's evolution. If he controls one stream of tendency today, tomorrow there is another stream; that is because not only is he open to invasion from outside but the entire past is there. The direction, the line of sensations, thoughts, emotions and impressions has been determined by our past, not only in this birth but in many births. So the problem that calls for solution is complex.

How man, the puny being that he is, can be expected to meet the situation is a relevant question. But, as you are aware, in this yoga of transformation one does not proceed alone. It is impossible for man unaided by a higher power to put one step forward. The seeker can prepare himself by way of purification, rejection, and surrender, but for the actual working out of the change he needs a higher impetus, a higher dynamism.

With these provisos, when he starts he has to lay equal emphasis on the mind, the heart, the will. The traditional way of emphasising only one aspect of the personality to the exclusion of others is not open to the sadhaka of the Integral Yoga. In the traditional yoga of knowledge it is enough that the seeker uses his discrimination to separate the true from the false, the eternal from the transient, that he looks for Brahman, the Divine Reality and concentrates only upon it. He ignores all other things, he ignores his whole being except the concentrating mental faculty: the heart dries up, the life-energies are bottled up, the physical body is left to itself—they are of no concern to the seeker of the path of knowledge. Similarly, in the traditional yoga of devotion the seeker is concerned with the opening of the heart to the presence and influence of God as love, harmony, beauty. He shuts himself from the riches of the mind, from the dynamism of life. So too in the yoga of action, the seeker does work disinterestedly, but work and nothing else. He is not concerned with the illumination of the mind, with the emotional richness of surrender to the Lord. But in the Integral Yoga all these centres demand attention.

One may start in the particular area where the nature is most developed, where one is most ready by temperament and equipment. Each one of us has a different starting point but that shall not be the final point. One has to have the total view; the gains in one centre have to be communicated to the others.

Sri Aurobindo points out that one has to learn to concentrate upon the One, the sole Reality that exists in the universe. Everything must point to Him, to That. The whole mind must be soaked with the idea and truth of oneness, of God. But that is not enough. Simultaneously the heart must be opened, it must be trained, it must be cultured to embrace the Divine in the All—the Divine is not merely one and sole but all and multiple. One has to first mentally conceive that the Divine is in all and then learn to respond, to vibrate to the felt presence of the Divinity among all. The mind concentrates upon the One, the heart expands and embraces the Divine in the All, and the will presiding over the energies subordinates itself to the Divine Master and learns to effectuate whatever impulse is imparted to it from within or from above.

In this context, Sri Aurobindo notes that it is not enough to have a mental knowledge. This knowledge is necessary—to know what is and what is not is indeed indispensable, otherwise one does not know where one is—but to know from books and from others who have had the experience, to know mentally, is only the starting point. Unless mental knowledge is translated into living practice it remains dry learning, it is not an effective force for yogic or spiritual evolution.

One cannot, either, limit the realisation to a particular aspect of the Divine chosen by the mind. The Divine has many facets and poises. The seeker conceives and approaches the Divine as a Supreme Master, as a Supreme Lord to whom he surrenders his whole being, but he is also aware that the Divine is not limited to the personality of his conception. There are vast impersonal poises through which the Divine is spread and manifest (let us not at the moment speak of that part which is unmanifest): existence, consciousness, bliss. These impersonal realities, these states of being, consciousness, and delight belong to the Divine Being. Personality and impersonality are parallel truths, the obverse and the reverse of the same Reality. The seeker keeps his being open to whatever experience or realisation is vouchsafed to him. He does not determine beforehand the form in which the realisation should come.

He uses, to start with, the lever which Nature normally employs in day to day life: desire is the motive force of action in this world of lower nature. The seeker starts at that point, he turns his desire from worldly

pursuits to the single pursuit of the Eternal, of the
Divine. Desire as an incentive is turned towards God;
things start with great enthusiasm. Gradually as he
progresses and as higher and more veiled states of being
are opened, he learns and begins to transfer the very
poise of desire, he gives up the initial standpoint of desire.
He seeks perfection and liberation not for himself but
for the Divine. All are part of a divine scheme, each
man has a part to play. It is as a part of the divine creation, it is to manifest the Divine and participate in that
creation, that liberation from ignorance, a kind of perfection in spiritual consciousness is aimed at. The basic
perspective of the desire is changed in that he no more
seeks liberation for himself but for the Divine. The third
step is when he learns to work and anticipate not in the
way he wants but in the way that is indicated. He does
not determine beforehand that yoga shall go in this way,
in that direction, but allows himself to be wafted in the
manner and in the direction chosen by the almighty
Grace.

Necessarily, this training and conversion of desire is
accompanied by stages of self-surrender, which itself
also passes through three phases. The first stage of self-
consecration—self-consecration means the working out
of the central determination to surrender in day to day
detail—is characterised by intense personal effort. One
summons the best of oneself and seeks in every way at
every moment to submit to the higher guidance and
force. As a result of this constant, burning aspiration and
exertion of will, there begins a response from the Divine:
it may be from here [gesture pointing to the heart-
centre] or from above. It answers, it gives support
to the aspiration. And there is in the second stage a
mixed or joint endeavour in which the upward aspiration is constantly seconded and supported by a descend-

ing grace or spiritual force. The third stage is when the whole of the personal effort has been assumed by the divine working. The personal element loses itself and becomes no more than a channel for the working of the divine force. These are the three stages of surrender: personal effort, effort constantly seconded by the higher descent, purely a divine working.

Necessarily, the stage of personal effort is the most important for the seeker till he learns to dissolve himself, to be dead to himself. As long as the ego is active and ambition is present, the shadow of ego prevails and personal exertion is indispensable. It is only after the ego is surpassed that the sadhana can be said to be taken up by the higher yogic power and one need not make a personal effort; though one has to put in the labour of vigilance, receptivity, and a constant response to the action of the higher or the deeper force.

In what way surrender to the Divine is to be worked out, first in action on the physical plane, is the subject of the next chapter.

4

SELF-SURRENDER IN WORKS

A very potent mantra has been given by Sri Aurobindo to invoke the Supreme Divine Mother:

OM anandamayi chaitanyamayi satyamayi parame

Like all traditional mantras, it begins with the symbol *OM,* which stands for the pervading Reality that cannot be expressed by any form, but whose vibrations are most nearly represented in human speech by this syllable. By repeating OM you invoke the primal Reality and link yourself with it in the depths of your being.

Then comes *anandamayi,* blissful, it is a rising movement. When the human soul rises beyond the triple world of ignorance, the lower hemisphere, and enters into the higher hemisphere of the spirit, the first worlds that greet it are the worlds of bliss, ananda, delight. That is why the first invocation is for the Mother of Bliss. A causeless delight is there. It is a world full of the seas of delight. The Divine Creatrix is present as the blissful power and greets the seeker in that form.

The soul that is not content with realising the bliss, ascends further and is greeted by a deeper aspect of reality. One realises that what one has experienced is not merely bliss but something which is deeply conscious, deeply aware, something which is cognisant, self-aware and all-aware. The creative Puissance reveals herself as full of consciousness, as made of consciousness, as one whose nature is consciousness—*chaitanyamayi.*

The adventurous soul climbs still further in the heirarchy of the worlds of manifest creation. It comes across the vastness of the sheer truth-existence. Neither the Divine's nature of consciousness nor its expression as bliss is felt. One is aware of a sheer existence of truth. That is the Divine Mother as truth existence.

Even this summit, the three worlds of delight, consciousness and truth-existence, does not exhaust the being, the reality that is the Divine Mother. She transcends. There is still a beyond. She is free from her self-formulations in the triple worlds of the higher hemisphere. She is supreme. And it is to this transcendental aspect of the divine Puissance, the creative Force, that the last word, *parame,* supreme, is addressed. To the adorable Mother of all creation, let us offer our salutations.

And it is our good fortune that all these four aspects of the divine manifestation, all these four poises of the Divine turned towards manifestation, are embodied in her who is our Mother and in whose *mandir,* consecrated chamber, you all have the privilege to work. At one and the same time, she exists on all four levels. Present as the Mother of Bliss, looming above is her personality as the Mother-Consciousness, behind as the Mother of Truth, and over all as the Supreme Mother. All four are simultaneously present.

No great achievement, no consummation of yoga is possible—at any rate in this yoga of integral perfection —without a complete surrender to the Divine Mother. And surrender is a big term. Someone once said to me: " It's very easy, if we just surrender, the Divine is obliged to do everything for us. There is no other sadhana." I pointed out that surrender itself is a life-long sadhana. When I say I am surrendering, it is nothing more than an expression of an honest intention to surrender myself.

It is at best a will in my mind supported by aspiration in the heart to surrender. But there it may remain. Unless this determination to surrender is worked out moment to moment, from plane to plane of my being without respite, surrender remains a theory. How and in what part is one to surrender? That is the question.

As you are aware, this is a yoga which has reference to all the parts of the being. That being so, the call of surrender applies to the mind, the will, the emotions, the life-force, and even the physical body which has to learn to familiarise itself with the climate of surrender and establish its principle in the very cells. And Sri Aurobindo tells us that the one field where surrender can be worked out most easily and effectively is life itself, which includes all the dynamic expressions of our being. On the earth, life-experience is the chosen field. Even for one who does not do yoga, it is experiences gained in life—experiences chosen or visited upon one—that, in their accumulation, contribute to growth. The outer being participates in so many contacts, receives so many impacts and it suffers, rejoices, enjoys and goes on plodding. But all the while the inner monitor, the soul, derives the sap of that experience—not always in terms familiar to the external being but in its own way. It draws the sap, the *rasa* as we put it in India, and grows. For ages and ages the soul grows, in birth after birth the soul draws the essence of the experience of the outer being and forms itself, builds up a personality that gradually approximates and eventually reaches the godhead.

Yoga is a process of speeding up this development. We do not leave it to Nature to work out leisurely the evolution of the soul into its godhead. Yoga is a select means of accelerating the process of the divine unfoldment of the soul, the manifestation of the divine

consciousness in the human being. For this purpose, life
has to be seized at its very roots, the surrender has to be
applied in daily life. In the average person, nine-tenths
of life-activity is governed and impelled by desire. Desire
has many disguises. It is not always a naked desire, it
may work under the respectable camouflage of altruism,
philanthropy or duty. One should have the honesty to
recognise desire in whatever form it operates.

And the first cardinal condition for effecting the
surrender in Integral Yoga is to renounce desire. One
should make up one's mind not to work impelled by
desire or to choose work under its stress. One should
understand that—particularly in an environment like
this presided over by a Divine presence—the work that
comes to one is precisely what is most suited for one's
development. No personal preference, no mental con-
struction or formation should influence the individual
seeker in choosing work. The choice is to be left to the
Divine.

Once one has this free and open attitude to do
whatever work comes, the next important step is to
renounce the desire for the fruit of work. It is this desire
that creates impatience, fevered effort, fatigue and loss
of energy. Every moment that we work under the desire
for a particular fruit, one eye is turned towards that and
is also watching for any obstruction. One part does the
work but the other three-fourths is looking ahead at the
expected result. This leads firstly to fatigue. I remember
the Mother saying once that the ideal way to work is to
live in the moment. Live in and do the work that comes
to you at the moment. Don't think of the next moment,
don't look ahead for what is going to happen. If one
can take that attitude, much of the fatigue can be
avoided.

Secondly, when one does not tie oneself to the expectations of a particular fruit, there is no tension. There develops a sense of equality. Whatever comes is taken as the will of the Divine. To work is man's part, to give whatever result is the Divine's part. Renunciation of desire for the fruit leads to the natural growth of an equality of action. And this spiritual equality in yoga is different from an attitude of indifference, a stoic fortitude or lack of interest. Equality means an unperturbed reception of what comes to one, an equal readiness to accept whatever is given, a vision and poise of equality when meeting others. This quality has necessarily to be cultivated from the outset. As it establishes itself, it develops into a great power which works spontaneously. But till then, equality has to be assiduously fostered. With the stabilisation of equality, there is an erosion of the divisions of the ego. The ego is normally concerned with personal aggrandisement, with exploiting every situation for personal gain, but once the desire for the choice of work and the fruit of work is abandoned, the ego loses a strong foothold. With the weakening of the ego, there develops a sense of oneness with one's fellowmen. The divisiveness of the ego is weakened. The doors are opened for the realisation of the eventual oneness.

It may be asked, if one is not to exercise a personal choice in work, if one is not to expect a particular fruit in work, is it possible for human beings to act with interest, or will work then be done merely in a mechanical way? Work under these conditions ceases to be work in the ordinary sense. It is uplifted to a sacred dimension. Work is converted into a sacrifice. It is an occasion for the outpouring of one's energies to the Divine Master who governs and to whom we are making an effort to give ourselves. Work becomes a means of approaching the Divine in a concrete way. It is a means for growth. With the development of the right spirit, work forges a channel for the upflow of the consciousness towards the Divine. It also acts as a channel for the downflow of the divine peace, strength and consciousness into the human vessel.

Man begins by becoming a conscious instrument; he is aware he is the doer but he works for the Divine. The second stage is when he learns to drop the doer in him, to tune himself to the divine power which is really the worker in the universe. He converts himself into a channel for the working of that *shakti,* of that divine power. From an instrument, he converts himself into a channel, proceeding in his effort so to be as wide and conscious a channel as possible. There develops in him a certain identification with the power that flows. Love, devotion, self-giving all have their own contribution in enlarging the area of his identification with the Divine Shakti. The final step is when the worker ceases even to be a channel but becomes one with the universal power that works. He is no more than a point of radiation. He has no separate will. His will becomes a fulcrum for the operation of the universal will on Earth.

Sri Aurobindo refers with great feeling to the Bhagavad Gita as the first broad statement of the doctrine of works ever given to man. I do not know how many of you are aware that it has played a remarkable part in the spiritual life of both Sri Aurobindo and the Mother.

To those of you who are not familiar with the topic of the Gita, I would first mention in brief that it purports to be a discourse between Lord Krishna, the avatar of the age and Arjuna, the fighting prince in the

Mahabharata war who represents man. On the eve of
the decisive battle, when both the hosts were assembled
and standing ready to enter action, Arjuna, who was
leading the forces of the righteous princes, sees in the
opposite camp his own teachers, sires and relations whom
he is called upon to kill. A false sense of pity and compassion comes over him, he drops his bow and arrow
and tells his companion charioteer, Lord Krishna, that
he will not fight. It is then that Lord Krishna begins a
discourse which runs into eighteen chapters, covering
the gamut of spiritual life. The main theme is the gospel
of works; man has a duty to God which is much more
than his duty to his family, country or fellowmen. It
is a vast subject which we shall not now enter into, but
karmayoga as it has been known all over the world has its
basis in this dialogue between Krishna and Arjuna.

The Mother has said in one of her conversations
that during her younger days in France there was a crisis
in her inner life and she did not know which way to turn.
She wanted very much to know something of the Eastern
spiritual wisdom and she was waiting. It was then that
an Indian patriot who happened to be there placed in
her hands a very unsatisfactory French translation of an
English rendering of the Gita. And the Mother has
described how much she benefitted from that contact
with the Gita. She had occasion to mention this incident when she remarked that in the Ashram we take
things for granted—we don't have to struggle for spiritual guidance. We don't have to make the effort, do
the *tapasya* to get spiritual knowledge as the ancients had
to, as even Mother and Sri Aurobindo had to. It is
given for the asking; we have only to receive it. And she
remarked with a certain poignancy, things are available
but eyes are turned elsewhere.

When Sri Aurobindo was in the Alipore jail for a full year imprisoned under false charges, he studied the Gita deeply. During this period he had the experience, the revelation, of the universal godhead, Vasudeva. Vasudeva means the God who is everywhere, Krishna who is everywhere. He saw the universal Lord around him, above him, in everyone, and everywhere.

I have been collecting for a small book all the Sanskrit references in Sri Aurobindo's writings in English and tracing them to their source in the various Sanskirt scriptures or classics. And to my amazement, I find that at least fifty to sixty per cent of his citations are from the Gita. That will give you an idea of its importance.

There have been hundreds of commentaries on the Gita from various points of view and still today people are writing. It is a living fountain of spiritual inspiration. But the exposition that is most suited to the modern mind and most helpful for gaining an entry into the intricacies of the Integral Yoga, is Sri Aurobindo's, *Essays on the Gita*.

Any questions?

Would you elucidate the conception of swabhava *in the context of yoga?*

When one is purified of the sediment and film of lower nature, the real swabhava, the real mould of the being, comes forward and you become aware of your true field of action, the true way of your growth. Things are not determined by birth or heredity; in spiritual life at any rate, it is the swabhava of the embodied soul that should be the deciding factor. As the society declined, the swabhava came to be determined by the particular class or caste in which men were born. But that is not

what it was in the earlier ages of India. Only the teacher
could determine the real swabhava of the individual and
prescribe to him the particular sadhana that could take
him to his heights.

In the Integral Yoga we have to orientate our
nature to the goal, in the direction of the goal. Viewed
from a deeper angle, each man has four natures, not
one. Just as there are four powers of the Divine Mother,
there are four powers of the human personality. It will
not do for one who seeks integral perfection to arrive at
the perfection of the knowledge element alone, nor the
perfection of the heroic, the harmonising and productive,
or the service elements alone. All four have to be forged
into a whole.

The Gita represents a certain stage in the development of human thought. Much has happened thereafter.
The concept of the supramental consciousness, the gnostic light, is not in the Gita because the human mind was
not ready for it. Each scripture gives just what aspiring
humanity is ready for and a little more, so to pull it
further. Each age has a scripture, but scripture of the
past has always a message for the man who is psycho-
logically at that stage.

*Can we say that in karmayoga each work ought to be done
with indifference and an attitude of surrender?*

Indifference, no. Work has to be done with interest.
Indifference applies to the results.

*What I mean is indifference to the type or nature of the
work.*

All work is sacred. It is a mental notion that one
work is superior to another. All work entails an outpouring of energies at whatever level it may be—mental,
vital, physical. This outpouring of energies must be a

sacrifice to the Divine. Whether you write a book or clean a floor, when it is done as an act of consecration there is a growth of the inner consciousness. If you are just a mental thinker, you can write a hundred volumes and your consciousness may not grow spiritually— mentally it may form itself, but spiritually it may not develop at all. Whatever you do, each work is an occasion for the culture of the consciousness through self-consecration.

Is it not true that working in a place like the Matri-mandir can itself prepare one to work in the yogic spirit of consecration?

That is true. Certain works have a special significance. But only those who are ready to take advantage of that situation can benefit from it. Even if one works at the Matrimandir, if it is in the normal egoistic spirit it won't help; though perhaps the vibrations may indirectly awaken one at some time. It is a question of attitude.

Such favourable circumstances, such specially charged environments, are provided for souls who are ready to gain from them. Just as there are on earth concentrations of beauty or power, so too there are concentrations of spiritual energy. Though in essence all is one, all is God's manifestation, in expression there are deliberately designed concentrations. And to these points chosen souls are attracted and brought so that they may take the lead and be uplifted. I have no doubt that the Matri-mandir is one such capital concentration of power, giving a vast opportunity to aspiring souls. Here especially, it is not just work. I agree that with a spirit of dedication and surrender, one will always gain more here because the concentration of forces is different. But it is not everyone who is circumstanced to work here.

Are there other true indications besides the joy of creation
to show that one is on the right path in the yoga of works?

Yes; there is no fatigue. Of course if you work too
much there is a certain physical fatigue, but otherwise
there is none. And there is no sense of time. One is
carried as in a stream. There is an ebullition of joy and
there is no fatigue. Mother says that when there is
fatigue, look into yourself and see why it is there and see
where you have failed to have the right attitude.

5

THE SACRIFICE

We are told in the scriptures that at the commencement of this creation, having created man, the gods and the rest of the universe, the Lord commanded: "With sacrifice for companion you go forth in the world; by sacrifice you foster yourselves."

Sacrifice is one of the great fundamental truths of life in this creation; its fuller significance becomes patent to us in spiritual life. Indeed, sacrifice as a truth obtains on every level of creation. It is Nature's means of rebuilding the unity of life which has been broken into fragments in the course of involution. Sacrifice is an interchange, a giving up of oneself to another, bridging the gulf that exists normally between any two in creation. It is understood that at lower levels of creation, sacrifice is more or less imposed; it is not voluntary, it is a compulsion of Nature by which each creature shares its life with others. At the human level, the principle of sacrifice is a corrective to the developing ego which tends to regard its temporary division and separativity as the sole, sufficing truth of life. Having been fragmented at the material level, creative Nature on its return journey brings in the law of interchange, of mutual self-giving, mutual help.

At first this working is disguised under whatever pleas, mental or vital. Men may think that they are associating themselves for their own safety, giving themselves to others in order to ensure their own self-existence. But the truth is otherwise. No man can live by himself. There is nothing in fact that belongs to oneself—the

physical body is derived from universal Matter, the very
breath it draws from the universal force of Life, the bit
of mind that is active in man is a fragment projected
from the universal Mind, the soul is a speck of the vast
Spirit manifest in the universe. This being the truth, it
is inevitable that each individual has to associate himself
with others if he is to forge a line of progress. Whether
he consciously wills it or not, an incessant interchange
goes on. For nourishment he draws upon the universal
physical- and life-energies and thought-forces that are
abroad, and he radiates constantly his own physical aura,
vital energies and thought vibrations. He pours them
out, rather they are poured out whether he is aware of it
or not, into the universe. Yoga seizes upon this central
truth of sacrifice or interchange at the origin of creation.

In response to the call of Nature, of the soul which
had lost itself in the depths of inconscience, the Divine
Light, the Supreme Grace plunged down at the sacrifice of itself and took its lodging in the darkness of matter
in order to reclaim the soul. In yoga too, there is a descent of the Divine Consciousness invoked by self-giving
on the part of the soul which has surrendered itself to its
master. The Divine responds to the human call.

And this readiness of the Divine to make a holocaust of himself, a sacrificial offering of himself, is the
heart of the doctrine of redemption. Man can be saved,
the world can be saved, because the Creator is ever-
ready to sacrifice himself for that purpose.

The sacrifice goes on at all levels. The sacrifice
between man and God is man sacrificing himself and all
that he cherishes, all that he has and contains, and the
Divine sacrificing its peace, its absoluteness, its supreme

consciousness, taking on itself the cloak of ignorance in order to help man to rise above the belt of ignorance.

It is this truth that has to be kept in mind. When one sacrifices oneself, apparently it may look as if one gives to the family, to the country, to humanity. But in fact, whatever the motive on the surface, he who receives is the Lord, the Divine. The Divine dwells in each form, in each creature, and once a true sacrifice is made in a spirit of consecration, it is the Divine in the object of sacrifice which responds and receives the sacrifice.

"As men approach Me, so I accept": that is the master-word of the Gita. The giving, the self-giving which is the key of sacrifice, may be through any form— a cup of water, a flower or a leaf, a thought, an emotion —but whatever the form, the Divine dweller receives it with a sacred regard. The point is, a spiritual seeker should become more and more conscious of this inter-change, of this self-giving. If for an ignorant man sacri-fice is forced by Nature, by circumstances, it behooves the awakened man to become conscious of it, to add signi-ficance to it, to become fully aware and make the sacri-fice consciously.

This after all is the meaning of that historic legend of the Brihadaranyaka Upanishad in the days when kings and sages ruled the hearts of men. King Janaka was governing the vast territories of an opulent king-dom, but at heart he was a master yogi. He ruled a kingdom, but he had also conquered the kingdom within himself. It is said that once when he was sitting listen-ing to words of wisdom of the sages who had gathered, a messenger rushed in saying that the capital, Mithila, was on fire. The king did not stir; he did not even look at him. The messenger repeated it once, twice, seeing

Janaka's imperturbability. The king finally turned round
and said even if the whole of Mithila were burned,
nothing of him could be singed.

At the court of this sage-king there was another
sage. He was not a king but a master of kings. Yajna-
valkya was his name. One day, so the story goes, he
decided to give up his possessions and retire to the forest.
He was a self-realised man but in keeping with the cus-
tom of those days he had two wives, and before retiring
he wanted to distribute his possessions equally between
them. He called his first wife, Maitreyi and said "I have
decided to retire, I will give you half of my possessions."

She replied by asking, "Will all the wealth that
you would give me assure me of immortality?"

He said, "Certainly not, it will give you all that
wealth can give, but nothing of immortality."

"Then what shall I do with the wealth that you
would give me? Instruct me in that which will give me
immortality; instruct me in the knowledge that will give
me the truth; I do not care for your wealth."

The sage was very much pleased and said, "Give
me your ear, I am very pleased that you have spoken
what you have." He then began a discourse emphasising
the uniqueness and the truth of the Divine Self which is
the sole truth in the universe.

He said that life is dear not because of life but
because of the Self that is manifest in life. The husband
is dear not because of the husband but because of the
Self. The wife is dear not because of the wife but because
of the Self. This important statement has been mis-
interpreted and perverted by commentators who have
given the meaning that one does not really love one's

wife because of her but for one's own selfish purposes. Well, it may be true at a certain level of life for certain individuals or as a general rule where the ego predominates that the spouse is dear for the sake of the lower self. But it is also true, and more true, that the wife is dear to the husband not because she is his wife, he is dear to her not because he is her husband, but because the Self, the central being, the Divine being that is *here* is also *there*. The Self in me recognises the same Self that is in another body, in another embodiment. There is a flow from the Self in one form to the same Self in another. There is a natural attraction because there is this interchange behind the surface. All is dear because of the Self. All moves towards this Self. When one sacrifices, it is to the Self that is within; the Self is the adored one to whom the sacrifice is made.

This doctrine of sacrifice was made the central truth of life by the ancient seers of the Veda. The rishis of the Veda were great mystics whose first concern was spiritual—not the spiritual as divorced from the temporal and the secular, but as both the high point and sustaining base of all that is in the universe. The rishis built sacrifice as the main institution around which they organised their individual and collective spiritual life.

They speak of the altar on which the sacrificial fire is burnt; necessarily they have to speak in images devised by human language. But the truth, as Sri Aurobindo has perceived and pointed out, is that the altar is the heart, the inner being, the purified chalice of the heart; the fire that burns is the flame of aspiration. One aspires intensely putting all that one has into that intensity and the flame shoots up calling the Divine, calling the Divine powers to come. The aspirant gives what he has; and when the offering is described, for example, in the

images of cows and horses, it really means he gives whatever knowledge and power he has acquired, whatever
occult power he has gained. Whatever the form, he
sacrifices all to the Divine Agni, the flame-power.

And as a means to render the mystic flame active,
the rishi recites the potent Word. These word-forces
are the mantras which, when properly intoned, release
certain vibrations in the physical and the subtle atmos-
pheres that invoke the presence of the gods. The Mother
has recorded somewhere that long before the Ashram
was formed Sri Aurobindo was explaining the Veda
to her, and when he recited the very first hymn to
agni, the mystic flame, she saw the flame concretely
before her. That is the potency of the Word.

As the rishi aspires, invokes the presence of the
gods and gives himself inwardly to them, the first to
appear is Indra, the god of the Divine Mind. Man is a
mental being and when he catches that fire of self-giving
it is the mind level that opens first to the higher mind
and becomes illumined—Indra manifests. Indra comes
with his force of Maruts, the storm gods which are the
thought-powers yoked to life. They are purified and
link man's energies to the illumined mind. Next to
appear is Varuna, the god of vastness. He is the lord of
the vast infinite. The being expands, breaks through
the walls of its ego. As said in *Savitri,* "the island ego
joins its continent". Once the being spreads out in the
vastitude of Varuna, Mitra comes, the god of love.
There is a welling out of the universal love, a love transcendent which breaks across the individual barrier,
which goes to the very root of creation and manifests
the Divine Love through the individual embodiment.
And there are many more gods who attend the sacrifice.
Suffice it to say that from the very beginning of the

spiritual development of humanity, sacrifice has been chosen as the one capital means of breaking out of the limits of humanity and linking oneself with the higher existence.

In the Integral Yoga, and particularly in the yoga of works with which we are concerned at the moment, sacrifice, the principle of self-surrender, self-consecration, plays an important part. Without it, work ceases to be sadhana, work becomes labour. Work has no spiritual significance, no yogic meaning, unless every bit of what one does is impelled by this feeling of self-surrender. One works for the Divine, one offers the work to the Divine.

As this spirit of sacrifice develops, one realises how silly the popular notions of sacrifice are. To the common man sacrifice means an increasing degree of self-denial, self-hurt, self-immolation. Actually, what is denied is indulgence; what is extirpated is the ego; what is released is the soul, the divinity within. In the Gita there is a significant chapter with a passage on the subject of sacrifice. The sacrifice in which man hurts and punishes himself, imposes hardship, severities and denials upon himself, is described by Lord Krishna as *asuric*, undivine. It is an offence against the indweller; it is a chastisement, a punishment of the Lord who is seated within. Instead, man is called upon to awaken his gentler faculties, his finer emotions, to summon all his powers of devotion and love and then surrender, then sacrifice, step by step. The Lord steps forth and receives the acceptable sacrifice.

This spirit of sacrifice is to be present not only in work but, Sri Aurobindo demands, through all the hours and activities of the day. Even when one eats, for example, one has to become aware that the food is being

consumed by the Divine within oneself. It has to be
accepted with gratitude from the donor, from the one
who serves the food, and offered to the Divine within in
a spirit of sacredness. So taken and so consumed, even
material food adds its own nourishment to the spiritual
well-being. There is an interchange even at the ordinary
physical level. The ancients even had a discipline by
which the act of breathing was converted by a mantra
into a beating of the universal heart of God. Each step
of the in-breathing and out-breathing was identified
with "I am He" and "He is I." The perception was a
living one. Each moment there was an identification
with the Divine, the universal Divine: "I am He, He is
I." This constant affirmation beneath the surface in the
very act of breathing made the presence so vivid, so concrete, that it left its impress on all the activities of life.

Sacrifice so conceived, so offered, so conducted, has
three results. Firstly, one cannot offer the sacrifice to
the gods, to the Divine, in a spirit of consecration unless
one puts all one's feeling and sincerity into it. Devotion
melts into feeling, feeling deepens into love; the love
regards the divine presence everywhere. Thus on every
occasion, in every movement, one feels the throb of the
Divine and it is a joy to consecrate oneself, to offer oneself, what one does and what one has to the Divine.

Secondly, one is always conscious of the liberating
knowledge that there is nothing except the Divine. All
that one sees is in the Divine; the Divine is in all; and
the all is Divine. This triple knowledge is a natural
truth-idea vibrating in the mind of the seeker of the
Integral Yoga who sacrifices to the Lord.

Thirdly, the human will for action and the will for
aggrandisement or gain is yoked to the higher purpose

of the soul. The very character of the will, the element of selfishness in the will, gets slowly dissolved and dis-associated from the personality. The inner will comes forward and replaces the egoistic will; and that inner will is nothing but a channel of the Divine Will.

There is, thus, a meeting of all the lines of yoga—love, knowledge, and will—in this integral path which proceeds upon a whole-hearted and illumined and loving consecration of oneself, of what one feels, thinks, does, hopes and aspires, to the Divine.

Any questions?

Is there ever an end to sacrificing for the Divine?

After a certain stage sacrifice ceases to be sacrifice. It is a happy interchange, it is a fusing of one into another, of the human into the Divine. That is the acme of sacrifice. And to the delight of fusion, of union, there is no foreseeable end. It is only in ignorance that there is an end of union. In knowledge, in light, there is no end to anything.

How does one distinguish between offering and sacrifice? Are they the same?

Offering is at the level of intention. The physical act of offering may also be present but basically it is an intention to give. But how far that intention is pure and clearly translated or is merely a mechanical giving of an object or a thought is another matter. Offering, when it matures into a spiritual quality, becomes the right sacrifice. It is like the intention to surrender; by merely deciding to surrender one does not surrender. One needs a whole lifetime to work out the discipline of surrender. So too sacrifice. It is a gradual, progressive discipline. But after a certain stage, it forges its own way. One does not have to exert oneself. One sacrifices normally as effortlessly as one breathes. Offering is the approach and sacrifice is the fruit.

What about the element of our weaknesses in the act of sacrifice?

Naturally the very act of sacrifice presupposes that *all* that you are and have is offered. But sincerely. Once you offer your weaknesses to the Divine, it is expected that you will follow it up by doing what the Divine expects of you. One has weakness, but in the very act of surrendering it to the Divine one receives the strength to get over it.

There are weaknesses which are beyond human capacity to overcome. They are best offered to the Divine in the person of the teacher or else directly. And here too the necessary strength is obtained to overcome the weaknesses. Once weakness is sincerely offered and surrendered, its roots are gone. There may be a mechanical indulgence in that weakness for a while but it loses its force if the offering has been sincere.

There is an increasing need on our part to recognise the Matrimandir as a consecrated area where a centre of the Mother is being built. Part of that movement is to offer the weaknesses of smoking of any kind, sex indulgence, etc. What would you consider a way of sacrifice to help build a collective effort in this direction?

An aspiration, a sincere aspiration that these atavistic elements must go from the atmosphere. A sincere prayer to help others to be free of these things.

And in the flame that is slowly building itself in the Matrimandir, all these weaknesses will be consumed. There is no doubt about it. In the very act of working, in the very act of serving, one releases certain forces, spiritual and occult, which will relegate these draw-backs to the background. They will just drop away. If as a result of certain karmic impressions or a fundamental insincerity the things continue, the person drops out.

It is always best and most profitable to emphasise the positive side of things and not look too much on the negative. As the positive gains gather, they simply displace the negative ones.

6

THE ASCENT OF THE SACRIFICE

Progress in and by sacrifice lies in inner consecration. The progress is in two directions. First, there is the growth in our nature of something that corresponds, in however small a measure, to the ideal which we seek and second, there is the revelation or the experience of the Divine in our inner experience.

To what extent one's nature is progressing is to be determined by each individual. It is a common question I am often asked: How can I know if I am progressing? And there is only one answer. If we are frank with ourselves, if we have the courage to face the truth, there is only one barometer: How do I react to men and things in day to day life? Is my reaction to events and people the same as it was before I took up yoga? If I react to anger or jealousy from another with the very same vibrations of resentment or anger, then certainly I am no different than he is. If, on the other hand, I see that there is a certain control and I do not respond to his vibrations but can detach myself and remain unaffected, that is an indication of one step gained. It is through our reactions to everyday events and through our thoughts, feelings, and actions that we can measure whether our nature changes or not, whether we are progressing or not.

The second element of progress is our inner experience of the Divine. The Divine that we seek, Sri Aurobindo points out, is not a monolithic reality; it is an infinite which is multitudinous in its manifestation. And the seeker of the integral reality has to keep himself open to an integral revelation. The revelation may come in one form or several forms simultaneously or successively. But the most important and basic perception that should form the foundation for other realisations is the awareness that behind all the fleeting phenomena of life, the changing forms and movements, there is something permanent, there is something eternal. Behind the turnings in time there is the Eternal that upholds these revolutions. Behind all the movements in the cosmos there is something which upbears the universe.

This perception and awakening to the existence of a Self, an irreducible Reality that does not pass but holds in its palms all that passes, is the base. We must at least mentally conceive, imagine, and link ourselves to this Reality. Once we establish the actuality of this eternal being and presence of the universe in our consciousness, there is a movement of liberation. We no more belong to transient phenomena. Some part of us has taken its poise in what is eternal, in what is basic.

That done, the first realisation and the easiest is to become aware of the divine presence within oneself. Very often it is asked: If the Divine is everywhere, why speak of it as dwelling within the heart? The fact is that while it is true that the Divine is stationed everywhere, it is more easily perceived within oneself. Awareness of this Divine Self in one's own heart leads to the awareness of the same Self in the hearts of others. You meet others on this base. This is the truth of Mother's saying that you can arrive at unity with others only at the soul level. Unity with others at any other level, emotional, mental or verbal, is an artificial unity. But if we touch the level of the Soul which is extended in all, we reach a point where we are one with others. To become aware of the divine presence within oneself, a presence not apart from the universe but dwelling in it, is one capital realisation.

A second, particularly for those who are naturally extrovert, is the perception of the divine presence without, in the world. This is also a mighty experience. Every form that passes before our eyes becomes a window opening on the divine presence in the universe.

And this is not all. We can awake to the Divine within ourselves, we can be aware and respond to the Divine outside ourselves in the universe, but there is also a third realisation which may very well press upon the seeker. One may realise the existence of a Reality which is not bound within the formula of the cosmos. It exceeds both the individual and the universe. Seen from that poise of transcendence, the whole universe looks like a speck, an individual a point, the entire movement a petty swarm. But Sri Aurobindo emphasises that this transcendent Reality is not to be looked upon as something divorced from the cosmos but as something that supports it, something that projects it, and yet it is outside its bounds.

These are the three major realisations that are open to the seeker of the Integral Yoga once he launches himself on the path of sacrifice. But in the course of the experience there are gradations; there are again, broadly, three lines of experience of the Divinity.

On one line he is conscious of a divine will, a divine presence in and around himself in the universe. It is eternal, ineffable, irreducible. But at the same time he sees that in the universe things are subject to time and limitation, things are not permanent, they are ephemeral. There is a constant movement and that movement is executed by a force, an energy which imposes the whole universe on his consciousness concretely. Some thinkers and seers have called this the power of *Maya*, the power of erecting a whole universe of appearances, forms and names on the pure being of *Brahman*. This is their experience, in appearance and concretely: the whole universe looks like an illusory phenomenon foisted on the pure white existence of Brahman.

This duality of the Brahman and Maya is the first to be met by the spiritual seeker on this line of development. But the true seeker does not stop at appearances. He goes deeper and finds that Maya is not merely a power that veils but it is also a power that creates; if it is a power that covers, it is equally a power that liberates. And it does not derive its power of creation from itself. It is a working of the will of Brahman, of the will of the creative personality in execution. If it appears to veil, it is because its processes are worked out in the field of ignorance. Once the seeker recognises this and looks up to the heights of knowledge, the same power of Maya works to liberate him from the hold of ignorance.

So the deceptive appearance of Maya as the sole creator and the power of illusion yields to the perception that the whole universe, the whole creation, is a projection of Brahman through its own creative power. This the ancients called Maya because in the older Sanskrit it meant something that measures, measures with cunning. The Divine Reality is immeasurable, yet a measurable universe is brought out of it. It is due to the existence of a power that has it within its ingenious working the capacity to project a finite out of a source that is infinite.

A second line of experience that the seeker comes across brings the perception within himself of a part that is aloof when he meditates, when he muses or is quiet. He feels a being within himself, the central being, that simply witnesses; it does not take part in the movement it perceives. The deeper the seeker delves into what is called the witness consciousness, he knows that there is a strong individualised conscious centre, the *Purusha*, who observes. And what does the Purusha observe? He observes a movement that is being worked out by an active energy. That energy is called *Prakriti*, nature. So here again there is a dichotomy, of soul and nature, Purusha and Prakriti.

If the seeker takes his stand in the witness consciousness he is aloof and not involved, he is liberated to that extent. If he loses himself in the revolutions of nature, of Prakriti, he is its slave; he is bound and there is no escape. But if he persists in going deeper he comes to see that nature works and moves in order to present experience to the soul. The soul regards, and in the very regard bestowed upon nature there is the assent.

Once he arrives at this perception it is possible to step from the position of slavery to the poise of mastery of nature by identification with the witness soul, which reveals itself to be a master soul at another level. It is then possible for the seeker to impose his conscious will on nature. The realisation of the Purusha and the Prakriti, soul and nature, is a second major experience.

The third line of experience that comes at a much later stage is the realisation of a Divine Soul within oneself—the Divine Godhead seated in one's being, governing manifestation—and of a Nature-power which is no longer ignorant but illumined, the *Shakti*. And the Shakti reveals itself to be none else than the active consciousness-force of the Godhead, of the *Ishwara*.

What began as *Brahman and Maya,* what pursued as *Purusha and Prakriti,* culminates in the experience of the *Ishwara and Shakti.* As was the case with the others, it is possible for the seeker to dwell primarily in the poise of either the Ishwara or the Shakti. Thus there have been seers who have dwelt more in the poise of Ishwara and looked upon the Shakti, the creative puissance, as something subordinate; and they have developed philosophies accordingly. There equally have been other seers who have taken their stand on the pedestal of the Shakti and have regarded the Lord as a passive witness, in effect, though not in theory, subordinate to the Shakti.

These three divine pairs reflect a fundamental principle in creation, the principle of polarity. The Divine Reality is indeed one, unique, alone. But when it chooses to manifest, when it chooses to bring out something from within itself, it assumes a biune expression. In the Indian tradition these have been expressively called the male and the female principles—-he and she. At all levels of the creation this dual principle is there, whether it is patent or latent. And even in spiritual life this principle of duality comes into operation at the level of manifestation.

There has been a good deal of misunderstanding on this subject particularly in Western quarters. I have seen scores of letters, read many books and talked to so many people that are under the delusion that every male spiritual seeker must have a "shakti" to arrive at fulfilment. This is an error and thrice an error as is its obverse formulation. A shakti, an instrument of creative puissance, is required only when the stage of divine manifestation arrives. And the stage for expression or manifestation of the divine glory is far, far off for ninety-nine percent of all seekers. One has to first develop the consciousness. One has to traverse a long way before one is in a position of having something to manifest. Till one arrives at a radical conversion of consciousness, if one believes that one has something to manifest, it is sheer egoism. It is not true. There is no necessity of a shakti or a Radha for a seeker.

And there is another occult truth which one must ever remember. This essential principle of polarity is instilled in every individual, whether he is a man or a woman. In each man there is a part that is feminine, in each woman there is a part that is masculine. It is possible to so arrange the workings of the twin principles within oneself that no outer instrument is necessary for manifestation—when that stage arrives.

Once the seeker is open to these varied experiences and revelations of the Divine, he ceases to be narrow-minded. He can only smile at the charges of poly-theism or the claims of monotheism by missionaries and propagators of philosophies and religions. Both views are in a sense true. For in certain lines of experience the uniqueness, the oneness, of God is preponderant. At another level the same One manifests himself in myriad figures, in multiple forms and allows himself to be approached through so many godheads. And the Divine manifests himself not merely through the many gods and goddesses, the many deities, but through all the million forms that are on the move—and those that are not even on the move—in the universe. An awakened seeker, and more so a yogin, regards the Divine in the smallest plant, insect, and stone.

This is the way and this the goal. The result is union with the Divine, which again can be of diverse kinds. The form of union which is most common to spiritual experience is union in the deepest Self with the

Divine by identity. I reach my soul level, the Self, and from there I identify myself with the Reality that is Divine; that is, in essence I am united with the Divine. This is called union by identity; it is attainment. In another kind of realisation the whole of my being, not only the core, dwells in the larger consciousness of the Divine. It always feels the Divine's presence to be close, initimately near. In a way, the being dwells in the world of the Divine. This indwelling in the realm of the Divine is a second type of realisation and union. The first type, by identity, is common in the way of knowledge; the second, dwelling close to the Divine breathing his air, is common in the way of love; there is a third. By training and discipline, by repeated consecration and orientation, the human nature grows into and puts on the higher Nature of the Divine. It bears resemblance to and it has the vibration and character of the Divine Nature. This is called similarity or likeness of nature. This is a rapid result of the yoga of works sincerely pursued.

Thus with all these realisations to be worked out, with all these types of union to be effected, it goes without saying that it is not only one part of the individual that progresses and merges into the Divine, but there is an ascent of the whole being towards the Divine. The mind, the soul, the heart, the emotions, the vital force, the body, and what is below—the whole being—is to be uplifted.

And the way proceeds in a series of ascents. There is not a single ascent but as the Vedic seer pointed out, one goes plateau by plateau. Each plateau brings before one the much more that is to be done, the large landscape that is still to be trodden. Each height reveals a new horizon. There are peaks after peaks that have

to be ascended. But, too, the integral seeker's is not
a one-way progress. Sri Aurobindo points out that for
each step taken forward and each ascending step scaled,
he must descend with the gain and relate it to the
rest of the being that has not yet participated in that
victory. He must integrate each gain with the rest of
the being. A series of ascents and a parallel series of
descents alone can work out the transformation of
nature.

And when this difficult process is pursued, one has
to fight not merely with the resistances and enemies
within one's own being, but one has to take account of
the enemies outside, the universal forces of resistance and
ignorance which are loath to yield the territory that has
been under their dominion for ages. All kinds of opposi-
tions, individual and universal, have to be conquered.
But no human individual, however strong, can hope to
do it unaided. And that is where comes the call for
surrender, the need for self-giving. One surrenders oneself to the higher yoga-force, the divine Mother-force
that oversees the whole spiritual endeavour of man.
One delivers oneself into her hands.

And the effective link between the individual here
and the divine power that works from above, is in the
emergence of what is called a *psychic being* within oneself. In philosophy it is loosely called the soul, though
there is actually a considerable difference between the
psychic and the soul; we will elaborate that distinction
next time. With the emergence of the psychic being
from behind the veil, half the battle is won. The Divine
thereby obtains a strong foothold to enable it to function
in the external nature to obviate difficulties posed by
the lower nature. Till this emergence, the assent of the
mind, the emotional and the vital beings, and the body

are all necessary. But once the psychic being emerges in the front and assumes active control of the rest of the being, progress upon the path becomes rapid.

I have received an interesting question regarding the psychic:

Sri Aurobindo says the mental Purusha *is a witness, not the controller and lord of nature; it is only when we rise to the* Vijnanamaya Purusha *that the true lordship prevails. Is the psychic a witness consciousness or a true lord of nature or something else?*

The psychic is not the lord of nature. The psychic is a presence. It acts and guides when it is consulted, otherwise it remains a witness. The psychic may prompt a nature from behind which is accustomed to be guided by it, even when its guidance is not sought. But if the promptings are ignored, once, twice, thrice, it falls silent. The psychic is not normally an element that imposes itself. It is a silent presence of the Divine which responds to our call.

The action of the psychic element also depends upon the stage of its development. The psychic essence, the psychic entity, the psychic being, are the several stages of the growth of the psychic presence. When it is a fully developed personality of the being, its functioning is something different. But in most seekers, the psychic is a silent presence which waits to be consulted, waits to be approached.

Due to the pressure of its instruments, the psychic often must submit to mistakes of action since it does not impose itself. When it does extend its guidance, that guidance is often immediately seized upon by the hungering vital or the interested ego and is perverted. Even then the psychic warns with a sense of some inexplicable uneasiness in the stomach or in the centre of the heart. But if ignored, it again withdraws. The psychic does not interfere.

The psychic is not the truth-consciousness. It is, we may say, a delegate in evolution of the truth-being above. It is a growing presence in the rounds of evolution, adding stature day by day. The soul in evolution is called the psychic being.

Another question which has been raised concerns certain difficulties, real or imagined, in the process of transformation or change of nature. There is a good deal of misunderstanding among Western psychologists and their Indian followers that it is wrong to suppress movements of nature like sex. Their view is that it upsets the system, throws one into unnatural move-ments, and impedes natural development of the soul. It is only a half-truth. Suppression of sex, for example, is wrong and harmful only if there is physical suppression but a mental indulgence continues. Cessation from the physical act of sex itself is not at all harmful. On the other hand, there is a profound philosophy, which I do not propose to elaborate now, which explains that not only is abstention very healthy but it develops the indivi-dual potential and capacity for transformation. If the mind consents to a denial and does not indulge, then it is absolutely safe. Whatever the kind of conquest—be it over the greed for food, sex, power or something else— the first movement is always holding it down, suppressing. Once one gets sufficient control by suppression, then rejection of such movements becomes relatively easy. Rejection is the aim, rejection is three-fourths of the process in this context, but one necessarily starts with suppression.

Before ending, I would like to read a paper which I think reflects something of a spiritual revelation on the part of the individual who has written it. It has had a great impact on persons who have heard it, and it occurred to me when I was reading the paper to Mother that I should share it with you all. It was written by a young and talented seeker, less than thirty, who arrived here in pursuit of his quest under unusual circumstances. He wrote a letter to Mother that he wished very much to write something to her but his head was full of so many things, so many thought-currents, that he could not express himself. His letter to Mother said:

" Here in the Ashram, one beautiful day is followed by an even more beautiful one. I am happy to be work-ing in a society that wants something more than matter and machine. I have many things to tell you but it is hard for me to put what I think into words. If you ask me a question, I would find it easier to express myself. I hope my request will not interrupt your peace. I always see the light of your skin and the brightness of your eyes. Your eternal servant."

I did not seriously expect Mother to take note of this request, but when she was listening to the letter, she suddenly opened her eyes and said, " Take down the question." I was very pleasantly surprised, took down her question, " Do you believe in a progressive world?", and gave it to him later in the day. Naturally he was happy. And almost the next day he was back with his reply:

" I have received your much desired question to which I now give answer. Yes, I believe in the progress of the world in spite of the many men who are deter-mined to detain it. The light, the flame of the new consciousness that Sri Aurobindo announced and you have brought, advances with certain and firm steps. No human can detain something which is beyond his simple earthly consciousness. A new morning is dawning and in a day not far off, all men on earth will recognise the Father and the Mother of the universe, incarnate in an Indian man that is the most spiritual, intelligent and wise man on earth and in a white woman of the youngest race, which as youngest leaped into space. Now, after a natural inexperience, we can begin to count on a youth that wants no more lies from neurotic politicians and from a psychotic society. Now they want the truth. I hope that in a day not far off, like me, all the youth of the world of all races, religions, ideals and forms, come to pay homage to the truth, the eternal Truth—you and Sri Aurobindo, Mother and Father of us all, God. I await your answer and, please, another question. Writing to you makes me feel well and now it is easier. Your eternal servant."

Mother replied: "It is very good, you are welcome here. Blessings." Then she gave another question: " Do you believe that the next step in evolution is the appearance of the Supramental race? Do you aspire to belong to the Supramental race?"

We will read his answer at the conclusion of our next meeting.

7

THE PSYCHIC BEING

The concept of the psychic being has received a
special treatment in the thought of Sri Aurobindo and
the Mother. The significance given here to the term
psychic being is not to be found in any other philosophy,
Eastern or Western. In the West the psyche usually
means the "soul or spirit" that is not patent to the eyes,
that is distinct from the body. Or it is the mind functioning as the composite centre of thought, feeling, and
action; this is something like a combination of what we
call the mental and vital beings. In India also the precise
concept of the psychic being is not contained in any of
the traditional philosophies. Though it may be asked
whether the psychic being, which plays such a central
role in the spiritual evolution of man, is not the same as
the *Atman,* the Self, the Soul, it is not possible to answer
simply yes or no.

To give an adequate idea of what the psychic being
means we need to consider the origin of creation. When
the Divine Spirit decided to manifest, the Upanishad
describes, a million sparks sprang out of the central
Fire, each spark being a portion of that Divine Spirit.
Each started out with a truth-idea to realise along its
own line of fulfilment. Now, these millions of emanations
from the Divine Spirit choose their own lines of manifestation, and each such spark stations itself at the head
of its line. In the philosophy of Sri Aurobindo and the
Mother, this central portion of divinity presiding over
the line of each manifestation is called the *jivatman.* It is
the Divine Self indeed, but the Self individualised for the

purpose of manifestation. You can imagine that there are millions of such individuations of the Self, yet the Self remains one. For purposes of creation or expression, it is formulated as so many centres of manifestation.

At the head of each manifestation—here we will consider only each human manifestation—there is, then, this jivatman. Standing above the evolution, it is not involved in it. It is presiding over the evolution of the truth-idea with which it is concerned from above. Now, in the course of evolution, the jivatman projects a small portion of itself, a deputy as it were, as a spark. This spark of the Divine Self that is presiding over it, is called the psychic essence. It is the soul substance. It can be imaged as a small ray which from birth to birth gathers about it the stuff of experience and develops a shape. Birth after birth gathering the sap of experience, the essence develops, puts on a shape, and gradually develops into an entity and then into a being. This evolution of the psychic essence into the psychic being is a fundamental part of human evolution.

Is there a difference between the soul and the psychic being? That part of the soul which participates in evolution is the psychic being. The part which does not involve itself in evolution is a witness, it holds itself aloof; that portion of the soul is not the psychic. The soul as involved in manifestation is the psychic being. The psychic being is never stationary; it grows, and to develop is its nature.

Where is it situated precisely? The psychic essence is at the core of the being. As an essence, one cannot feel the psychic as such, but one can begin to feel something when it acquires a certain individuality. The precise location is behind the cardiac centre, what is called the heart-centre in yoga. Behind the point of juncture of the vital from below and the mind from above, is the place of the psychic being. The psychic being may be called the growing Divine in the individual. Just as there is a distinction between the jivatman above and the psychic being within the evolution, a distinction has also to be made between this evolving divine entity in the human form and what the Gita describes as the Lord stationed in the heart of all creatures, who turns them round and round mounted on a machine by his Maya. That Lord is somewhere still deeper than the psychic. The psychic being may be looked upon as a living representative of the Divine Lord, but it is not itself the Divine Lord.

Now, what exactly does the psychic being represent, beyond saying that it represents the Divine? For everything on Earth, everything in evolution, represents the Divine. Sri Aurobindo has explained that just as matter is a projection, a representation of the sheer Existence above, just as the life-force is a projection of the Consciousness-Force, and just as the mind is a projection of the Supermind, the psychic is a projection of the Ananda, the Divine's principle of delight and love. The growth of the psychic is the efflorescence of joy, happiness and love. It is natural to the psychic being to be conscious of the parent Divine from which it derived. The psychic being always is the bhakta; devotion and love are as natural to it as breathing is to us. When a ray from the psychic reaches the surface of our external being, we are filled with a causeless joy, we become aware of the vast divinity around us, we begin to see something auspicious, something holy in others, to recognise the infinite in Nature around us.

When the psychic influence begins to take shape and organises itself increasingly in an individual, he awakes to the existence of spiritual life. Man begins to question and to be dissatisfied with the ordinary life he is leading; he wonders whether there is not a greater and deeper reality more satisfying.

For the spiritual seeker it is not the mind, not the vital, not the physical body, but it is the psychic element in him that is of paramount importance. Indeed the seeker does not need to awake the psychic being. He has turned to the spirit, he has taken to spiritual life, because the psychic is awakened and is putting its pressure upon his external being. What he has to do is aspire that more and more of the psychic influence may reach out to his being, may make itself present and felt. He has to exert his will and always keep one part of his attention turned inward towards the psychic, calling and drawing it out.

And the psychic always manifests itself in the values or in the powers of purity, harmony, beauty, joy, truth. These are not things to be taught and cultivated. Once the psychic influence begins to come to the front, these are things that come naturally; one spontaneously recognises the truth, feels the purity and rejects impurity, breathes out a causeless joy, emanates a feeling of one-ness and love towards all creatures. It stands to reason that when the seeker aspires for and calls out the psychic being within, it is incumbent upon him to create a milieu, an environment within and around himself that is conducive to the emergence of the psychic. Necessarily he has to eliminate from himself movements— mental, emotional, and physical—which are opposed to purity, harmony, happiness, goodwill, beauty. Any vestiges of ugliness, disorder or falsehood, repel the psychic light.

In answer to the aspiration of the seeker, the psychic being first sends its influence. The psychic being cannot emerge at once, it first sends its rays and exerts its influence to modify and shape the outer life. Sri Aurobindo describes this working in his great epic *Savitri*:

> Our soul from its mysterious chamber acts;
> Its influence pressing on our heart and mind
> Pushes them to exceed their mortal selves.
> It seeks for Good and Beauty and for God.

First it couches its influence in temporary rays; then as the outer being becomes purified and thus ready, the influence stays longer, a habit of psychic functioning is created. And it is only at the end of a long, long journey of personal self-equipment and development that the psychic being comes fully forward and takes charge of the spiritual evolution of the individual.

It may be asked if the psychic is indispensable for spiritual attainment. If there is only the question of the attainment of liberation, *moksha*, salvation, release from the world, indeed the psychic contact and influence is not necessary. The usual detachment of the soul, of the Self, is quite enough as the first and decisive step. But where there is the question of submitting the whole of human nature to the impact of transformation in terms of the Spirit, of transcending with the whole being the barriers of ignorance and falsehood, and growth into the realm of light and truth, the intermediary role of the psychic being is indispensable. The psychic being not only puts one in contact with the Divine Lord within but opens up the doors to the ascent above, to the higher realms of spiritual consciousness. It always gives the lead, it holds the light for the aspiring soul to scale the heights of the Spirit. And, as Sri Aurobindo points out,

the psychic being is a direct representative of the transcendent Divine on Earth. Its agency, its intermediary
role, is indispensable. He writes in *Savitri*:

> Earth must transform herself and equal Heaven
> Or Heaven descend into earth's mortal state.
> But for such vast spiritual change to be,
> Out of the mystic cavern in man's heart
> The heavenly Psyche must put off her veil
> And step into common nature's crowded rooms
> And stand uncovered in that nature's front
> And rule its thoughts and fill the body and life.

Thus far regarding the psychic being in the mi-
crocosm, in the individual. As in the individual, so in
the universe. Just as the psychic principle or being is
supporting from behind the veil the evolution of the
individual from the nescient to the superconscient, from
darkness to light, from death to immortality, through
countless ages, births and deaths, similarly, in the world's
scheme also it is the psychic world that supports the
terrestrial scheme. In the gradation of planes in the
terrestrial scheme of manifestation, there is the physical
world that we see, there is the life world which is not
perceptible, there is the world of mind. Now this triple
world in manifestation, the lower hemisphere as it is
called, is supported at the back by the psychic world.
It is in the psychic world that the evolution of souls, the
progress of evolving beings, is planned and directed.

The passage to that world is of interest. When a
man dies on Earth, first he sheds the physical body. He
lives in his subtle-physical envelope. After the time
which it takes for him to realise that he is dead, he looks
round and finds himself in a subtle world which is a
perfect replica of the physical world that he has left

behind. That is the subtle-physical world. Once he is
free of those pulls which hold him to the Earth—either
by way of his own desire or the pulls of grief or attachment of those behind—he leaves the subtle-physical
world and goes to the vital world. There it is a world of
desire. The karma that has been forged on Earth by his
vital being, the desires, sensations, ambitions, are all
found formed there. If they have been desires of the
higher type, he meets their renderings as heavens; if
they have been of the crude and ugly type, he is confronted by a veritable hell. He has to stay in the vital
world until, helped by the presiding powers, the vital
sheath is gradually thinned and drops off. Then he
goes to the mental world where he is surrounded by the
formations that he has woven by his thoughts, ideas and
conceptions. These also take time to dissolve. So after
all these sheaths—the subtle-physical, life, and mental
sheaths—are dissolved, the inner being, the soul, is free
to go to its place of rest and preparation, the psychic
world:

> The beings that once wore forms on earth sat there
> In shining chambers of spiritual sleep.
>
> .   .   .   .
>
> All now was gathered into pregnant rest:
> Person and nature suffered a slumber change.
> In trance they gathered back their bygone selves. ...
>
> .   .   .   .
>
> Arranged the map of their coming destiny's course:
> Heirs of their past, their future's discoverers,
> Electors of their own self-chosen lot,
> They waited for the adventure of new life.

This in brief is the role of the psychic principle in
the individual and the universal schemes.

Are there any questions regarding the psychic being?

How is one to be sure that an inner guidance is coming from the psychic being?

It is an experience of many that when they begin to live a kind of inner life, they become aware of a new personality within themselves, and it is very tempting to believe that this new entity is the psychic being. But in ninety-nine percent of the cases, it is not. The psychic takes a long time to express itself.

What happens is that once we withdraw from our external preoccupations, what we become aware of is either the subtle-physical Purusha, the vital Purusha, or the mental Purusha. These are inner selves, and each on its plane can appear to be the psychic being. One has to be extremely discriminating. If one hears a voice, there is always a temptation to feel it is the voice of the conscience, of the soul, of God. Those who believe indiscriminately that that inner voice is the divine voice, have invariably come to grief. There are voices and voices. Our own ego, our own preferences and mental constructions, have a way of voicing themselves; these are obviously pseudo-voices. For one genuine voice there are ninety-nine pseudo-voices. As well as in spiritual life, also in politics, in social affairs, in family matters, the pseudo-voice is to be guarded against.

People mistake the vital being, the mental being or any subtler formation for the psychic being. When the psychic emerges and begins to express itself, there is an unquestionable conviction it carries about it. There is a solid peace, a feeling of purity, an absolutely new dimension added. One knows that it does not answer to any personal preferences or desires. It is something fresh, at least for the moment when the psychic voice is heard; it is a new experience. But one has to be extremely discriminating, one has to be sure of one's purity and non-involvement in the problem, before taking the voice that one hears as a guiding voice.

A very interesting and practical question related to this has been asked of me:

When working with someone on a project and the guiding voice—which one believes to be the psychic—points the way, how should one proceed when the other party will not listen?

This is a question that faces most of us who are involved in a collective effort. I thought I should refer the question to Mother, so I read it out to her. She replied very emphatically: "Nobody is ever right *against* anybody." One can never impose one's own conviction, opinion or feeling on another. The right way for a seeker in a situation where there is a difference of opinion is not to believe that he is right and the other is wrong, but to submit the problem to the Divine in a spirit of surrender and trust. He can submit his own conviction and the whole problem and wait for the answer. In the measure of his sincerity, whether the other person is aware of it or not, the response does come and things do work out in the way they should, not necessarily as he believes to be right. One can never be sure that one is right. One is never right against anybody.

Naturally when working by oneself, one works to the best of one's light. There is a growing perception, and what was felt yesterday to be right may not feel as right tomorrow. But in a collective endeavour, the right attitude is to concede the freedom of others to follow

their own convictions. Where there is conflict or difference, submit to an overseeing power and await silently,
with trust, its guidance.

*When all those working on a common job live and are
guided by their psychic beings, to solve a problem will they each
simultaneously be pointed the way to the solution, or will they
be able to listen more inwardly on the mutual soul-level?*

I remember that the Mother once said long ago
that there is only one way of doing right, but there are a
hundred ways of doing wrong. So if all are open to the
guiding, the psychic, the spiritual light, naturally the
right solution and path will be indicated to all; but our
understanding, perception, and formulation of it in our
minds will necessarily differ. Here again it is a question
of conceding the right of each individual to progress and
contribute in his own way. One does one's best without
interfering with the growth of others, and leaves the rest
to the Divine.

When does the psychic assert itself?

As long as the psychic has not developed an individuality, it remains an influence which we accept or do
not accept. But once the psychic element develops into
a being and you are ready and make way for it, it assumes control and imposes its choice on the rest of the
being which is obliged to follow. When the psychic is
in front, there is no other choice except to be guided
by it. It dominates the whole of existence. Whether the
physical responds in its present state of formation is
another matter; but the psychic does indicate what is to
be done. It puts its seal and its purity even on the
physical, and makes it easier for the spiritual evolution
to proceed.

Is it safer to go to the astral worlds when the psychic is awake?

"Astral" is the Theosophical term for what we call the subtle or the vital. Naturally this and other planes become safer to enter when one is guided by the psychic light and has a psychic consciousness. When the consciousness is suffused with a psychic light, then what is called psychicisation takes place; it is then absolutely safe to leave the body, travel to the subtler, the astral worlds, have the necessary experience and come back. Otherwise for an unenlightened individual who is prisoner of his desires and sensations, it is dangerous to go voluntarily or involuntarily into the astral worlds.

We spoke at our last meeting of a young seeker who wrote to the Mother that his head was full of ideas but he could not express himself to her; he suggested that if Mother were to ask him a question perhaps he would be able to. Mother took note of his request, and asked him the question : " Do you believe in a progressive world?" His reply to this was read out to you last time. She then gave him another question: " Do you believe that the next step in evolution is the appearance of the Supramental race? Do you aspire to belong to this Supramental race?" Here is his answer:

" I received your marvellous statement and the two new beautiful questions, which I will now answer. Yes, I believe that the next step in evolution is the appearance of a Supramental race. What is more, I believe this race is here amongst us. All my being aspires to belong to this race; all that I am is laid on the Divine altar. The force, the light that exists within me, I feel is moving forward.

"I am not in a hurry, Mother; that light must go out. I don't believe in death, and I know I am something more than this body and this mind that cannot express all the love that I feel towards you, Sri Aurobindo and the world.

"Mother, my life has been a constant struggle against lies, and I always thought that he who lied to me lied to himself. The Divine answered me through you, the Divine Mother. Mother, I do believe in the new and great Supramental race, and I aspire to it with all my strength. I await your answer and the new question; it is so beautiful to speak in this way to you. Your eternal servant."

Mother remarked, "Let the Supramental Blessings be on you."

Her next question was, "Are you ready to silence your mind in order to be ready to receive the Supramental?" He answered:

"Four days ago I received your answer and even today I cannot find the words to express my gratitude for so great an honour. Your Supramental Blessings have fallen on me and opened new doors to the light, to the perseverance, to the struggle to arrive at the Divine goal which each day, and always with your constant presence, I see nearer.

"I will answer your new and as always beautiful question. Mother, I am ready to silence my mind; I do nothing else for some time. I love silence, the wonderful silence of life. I am awake, agile, fresh; there is no obstacle that can impede my surrender and my dedication to silence my mind to reach the goal. I conquer the forces of evil thinking of you, and *I don't know what failure is, since I have always seen it as experience.* [Emphasis added.]

" Mother, I had and have the flowers and the sun; now I have you in each cell of my body, in each movement of my wonderful daily life. I see you everywhere and in my dreams you appear also. I am ready to silence my mind and this way be ready to receive the Supramental. Mother, make me a torch of light and love.

" I await your answer and a new and always beautiful question. I always regarded life as beautiful, and how full of new light, hope and love it is now with you. I love you. Eternally at your feet."

Mother remarked, " This is excellent ", in reference to the phrase she underlined: " I don't know what failure is, since I have always seen it as experience." She was extremely pleased with this phrase which sums up a whole philosophy of life. Then she added:

> To live in the Divine,
>
> To work for the Divine,
>
> To plunge in the Supramental—
>> Blessings.

8

THE SACRIFICE OF KNOWLEDGE

We have thus far arrived at a conception of a reality that is integral in its character, that is the aim and object of our endeavour. We have seen that the reality is not merely an impersonal silence or power or consciousness, nor is it only a personality or a person familiarised by religion, nor is it just a state of being—but it is all of them together. The reality we seek, like the universe of which we are a part, has many aspects.

And since the reality has many aspects, our approach is also many-limbed. We approach the Divine not on one settled path, but on a number of paths, either simultaneously or one after another as the various folds of our nature open in the course of yoga. We have also discussed that the first door open to us, living as we do in the field of experience, is the one of sacrifice. Sacrifice not in the usual sense of self-immolation, but in the sense of self-consecration. And this sacrifice covers the whole of life. It is a sacrifice of our work, of our love and emotions, of our knowledge. And we mean by sacrifice not only the external aspect of the matter, the outer ritual and act of dedication, but more than this, the spirit within, the inner movement that backs up the outer act. When we speak of the sacrifice of works, for example, it means not only the external activities but all that goes on within us on the several levels of our being—the movements of the thought energy, the streamings of the emotional energy, the several formulations of the will.

So the sacrifice of Sri Aurobindo's conception embraces the whole becoming of man at every level, at every moment. The pouring of energies, outer and inner, is to be orientated towards the Divine not only in the beginning but from moment to moment. The dedication is to be affirmed, organised, and confirmed. If all the activities of our life are to be thus converted into offerings in the sacrifice to God, we are then to include even the day to day activities, insignificant as they look, inconsequential as they seem. The older traditions all over the world have demarcated activities as secular or religious: those which do not pertain to the soul's endeavour, those that should be severely left out, those that may be ignored, and those which alone are to be done and concentrated upon. Naturally, in our system, this divorce between the secular and the spiritual is not permissible. For the Divine is manifest in all the spheres of life, and the whole of life is our field. It is not merely a Beyond that is the proper field of the Spirit, but it is particularly the Earth that is the self-chosen field of the Lord. That being the premise, it is incumbent upon the seeker to embrace every aspect of his life in his effort; whether the activities appear to be directly connected with the spiritual effort or not, they have to be uplifted. Everything is to be informed with the guiding spirit, uplifted into a new dimension, and invested with a new significance.

It is thus unacceptable to follow the old injunction of the scripture that only those activities which strictly can be made a part of our religious or spiritual life are to be done and the rest gradually eliminated. This door of avoidance and escape is not open to us. The seeker of the Integral Yoga looks upon all activities as movements of the Spirit embodied in matter. All have their claim, all have to be cherished in the same spirit. As the Mother once said, whether you sweep the floor of a kitchen or perform surgery, the required attention, outpouring of energy, and dedication have to be brought to their highest pitch and consecrated to the Divine. It is not the act itself but the spirit that infuses it, the attitude behind the action, that ultimately weighs in the spiritual scale of values.

This does not mean that we continue doing the same thing in the same manner till the end of our time. Works have to be continued not only not in the same spirit, but after a time, not even in the same form. The level of the activity has to be gradually shifted upward and inward. The character of the work and the result vary according to the measure in which a new spirit, a new consciousness, is brought forward. If we do the work that we are obliged to do with the same mechanical mental attitude and spirit, we continue to move in the age-old rounds of ignorance. For that reason it is necessary that the endeavours to shift our centre of activity inward and the centre of our consciousness upward should continue simultaneously. With the opening of the being to the consciousness and light that pours from above, and with the assured support brought about by our contact with the inner soul, the psychic being, it is a safe journey. One has to open the daily programme of activity to the higher light. And each day one has to renew one's dedication, submit one's life activity to the higher light, and watch what changes take place in one's own consciousness and in the external field—whether the conditions and circumstances remain the same, get worse, or improve. These are measures of one's progress.

The seeker begins by offering in theory all actions to the Divine; there is a central determination of self-giving. The mind and will, the heart, and all the actions are offered; and to the best of one's ability they are treated to the inner and higher influence. Gradually, as the being finds its poise in the deeper consciousness, certain activities naturally fall away from the centre of the being. Those activities which tend to weaken the aspiration or obstruct the flow of the higher consciousness recede, and for a time the seeker confines himself to those activities which nourish his growth, which provide a rich field for the workings of that higher consciousness. But this is only a temporary, intermediary arrangement. In the third stage, as the higher consciousness gets stabilised, as the centre of activity gets firmly established in the psychic, the whole of life is gradually taken up and put in contact with the new consciousness.

This is the general background of the yoga of sacrifice. It is said that this yoga of sacrifice is to be applied in the three fields in which man is simultaneously active: the fields of knowledge, love, and work. Let us first analyse the sacrifice of knowledge.

There is the age-old distinction in India of human knowledge, of the outpourings of the mental seekings of knowledge, in two divisions: the higher knowledge and the lower knowledge. Or, as it is called in the Upanishads, the *para vidya* and the *apara vidya*. That means knowledge of the reality as approached and sought for from the lower material end, and knowledge that reveals itself from the higher end. The sciences, the various disciplines of knowledge and systems of thought that have been developed till now by the human mind—the Indian tradition speaks of as many as sixty-four branches of knowledge—are of the lower kind. They have been built by the evolving mind of man scanning the surface and probing the depths of things to analyse the truth of Nature and being. But the guiding light and principle is the mind. All these branches of knowledge constitute the

lower hemisphere of knowledge. But they are not, thereby, removed from the spiritual endeavour of man. They
are welcome to form constituents of the yogic effort.

If, however, in the vanity of its intellectual arrogance, the mind insists upon treating these branches of
lower knowledge as the final arbiters of truth, there it
utilises them beyond their legitimate range. Science, art,
and all these branches are valid in their own province.
They seek to probe into the processes of Nature, into as
much of the reality as yields itself on the relative surface
to the different approaches of the mind. But they are all
subservient to a knowledge that is greater than the mind,
a knowledge from which, as the ancient seers described,
"speech and the mind fall back unattaining". Literature, poetry, painting, music, architecture, and the
sciences are all so many windows on the reality that is
manifesting. But nothing more. Once we begin to live
the spiritual life of this conception, these subjects may be
studied, and some we are even compelled to study; but
we keep the proviso in view that they are subsidiaries to
a knowledge greater than the mind, a knowledge which
can be received by the mind in silence, reflected by the
mind in its purity, but which cannot be built by the
labouring intelligence. That knowledge is to be received
in the mind and being by purification, by opening to
ranges that open above the thinking mind. These are
ranges of the higher mind, the illumined mind, the
intuitive mind, the overmind, and even beyond to the
gnostic mind, the supramental consciousness. These
ranges are to be opened, and knowledge and light from
them is to be received, integrated in ourselves, and harmonised with our experience at the lower level. Our
experience and knowledge attained at the lower level
have to be corrected and set in proper proportion under

the pressure of the higher knowledge that descends. It is in this context that the sacrifice of knowledge is to be conducted. No knowledge is taboo, but everything has to be given its due value and nothing more.

People have asked Sri Aurobindo and the Mother if, for example, it is wrong spiritually to read novels or newspapers. Sri Aurobindo had no hesitation in answering that it is not wrong to read these or other things, all depends upon the attitude with which you do it. You may read the Gita or the Bible and yet remain the same degenerate man without being positively influenced. You can read any journal and yet keep your consciousness aloof and progressing. You read so as to take what nourishes and helps the growth of your consciousness at whatever level, and leave the rest. The consciousness shall not be allowed to dwell on any undesirable or unspiritual element that may be contained in a book, journal, or newspaper. If you are not strong enough mentally to keep out the undesirable element, then you should not read it; you should confine yourself only to what may be called safe literature. But a spiritual seeker of the integral reality is an intrepid adventurer, and it does not behove him to shut out this or that literature simply because it may upset him. He has to read what comes, understand and face the facts, reject what is not correct, but assimilate and benefit by what is offered to him. Very often when a book or journal is put in our hands unsought, it carries a message and has a meaning for us. We have to see why it has come. If we are not sufficiently strong to resist an unwelcome idea or an unholy association in a book, we are not really fit to be sadhaks of this yoga.

The other day a book was placed in my hand. A resident of Auroville asked if he could read the book consistent with his being a disciple of Sri Aurobindo and the Mother. The nature of the book is definitely mischievous. It is full of mixed knowledge, the kind of knowledge that was familiarised in the last century by a certain section of occultists. There is an element of truth, but ninety percent of it is imagination and vital mixture. So when I said that it was better not to confuse one's mind by reading it, the gentleman who had raised the question asked how as a spiritual seeker he could shut out some part of human experience which had been cultivated by an earnest mind. I could only answer that before using a book, one should have the discrimination to know what is to be accepted and what rejected. Very often the reader does not know. If a person who knows puts you on guard and you are discriminating enough, there is absolutely no harm in reading such a book. He was satisfied.

In any writing or branch of knowledge there is an element of truth and there is an element of error. There is no element of error in a knowledge which comes directly from the levels of the truth, from the truth-mind. But when something from there is taken possession of by the groping intelligence, when something is received even from above and immediately coated by the seeking mind, there is a great and definite possibility of error. This is something of which we must be aware. When I pointed this out to that gentleman, he asked if he could use the same proviso when reading the writings of Sri Aurobindo and the Mother. I said that he could, and added that Sri Aurobindo and the Mother never asked that their teachings or writings be taken on trust. It is for each one to read and confirm it in one's own experience. It is only initially that you start with a faith that Mother and Sri Aurobindo know something more than you do. No one asks that you accept Mother and Sri Aurobindo as Divine; no one asks that you regard what they have written as infallible truth. But as you can accept a book written by a physicist or a doctor as something said upon a subject which you do not know, here too that is enough. You start with a faith that there is something contained which you do not know; and if you are earnest, as you proceed the faith will extend itself. The knowledge that is given in the book will enlarge your consciousness in such a manner that the trust and the faith will gather. If there is a persistent resistance and hostility in you, it means that you are not ready for that truth, that truth is not meant for you and some other line of truth is open to and appropriate for you.

And incidentally, when you read the writings of Sri Aurobindo and the Mother—as indeed all authentic spiritual literature—don't ever try to understand or grasp with the mind. Have a receptive condition and read. Sail with the writing, don't try to understand or analyse. Just go along. As you become identified with the writing, something which is present in it leads you forward; it evokes a response in the heart and instills a calm and silence in the mind. And sometime later, well after you have finished reading, the sense will awaken in you. The Mother even said that when you read something written from the experience of a new consciousness, new cells begin to form in the brain to hold that knowledge content. It may reveal itself to your external being and consciousness much later. But you should keep up the effort of reading and not try to understand; the understanding will come in the heart and not in the head. Try this with *Savitri* or *The Synthesis of Yoga*. People say that the first canto in *Savitri* is difficult. But it does not matter if you don't understand; I have yet to meet a man who can confidently say that he has understood everything in *Savitri*. But this approach helps you to get into the spirit and adventure of the poem, and by the time you arrive at the last line, you are ready for the second canto.

There must be regularity in your study of spiritual literature. A fixed time has to be set for reading, because once you establish a regular time, the guiding spirit is present at that time hovering around you. You should make it a part of your sadhana to read these books as though they are spiritual food. We take physical food at regular times, and similarly this spiritual food also is to be taken in punctually. This truth of regularity, Sri Aurobindo has pointed out, is related to the truth of the natural rhythm in things. In God's manifestation there is at every level a rhythm, and we have to catch the secret of that rhythm and respond in tune with it. There is a rhythm of time, of consciousness, of movement. We have to build up a rhythm which can vibrate in tune with the universal rhythms that are ever active in the atmosphere.

Before asking for questions, I would like to consider a query or observation that I have received from a Matrimandir worker.

When any special work like concreting is in progress in this sacred place, it has been the experience of most of us that a special spiritual force is set in motion by the Mother and everyone feels its presence. One feels inspired and energised by the force, even has the visible experience of it, and is able to work with much more than one's normal capacity, with enthusiasm and elation.

It is a perfectly true perception. It has also been the experience of most of us in the Ashram all these decades that whenever there is a special function or work to be done and the Mother's attention is drawn to it, she does release a certain emanation which goes and presides, helping and guiding every participant in all ways for the execution of the work. But then the question is, why is it that just after the work is over one may feel hopelessly let down, tired and exhausted? I asked the Mother about this some fifteen or sixteen years ago. She said that when you begin to think of or look at yourself instead of being occupied with the work, the exhaustion and fatigue starts. If after the concreting or other work is over, you do not slacken and let the mind dwell upon yourself but become occupied with some other work, this exhaustion is not likely to appear. There has to be a tapering off. One shall not stop all activity the moment the actual work programme is over. One has to occupy oneself with something else and gradually lessen the tempo. Otherwise there is this feeling of sudden exhaustion because there is nothing, there is no will in us, to support the action of that force.

Questions?

How is one to balance the personal need for a regular schedule with the community's irregular work requirements?

There is also a rhythm between the elements of work, meditation, and study. And when there is a collective work there has to be a certain self-regulation and sacrifice of individual programmes. Priority has to be given to collective needs over individual ones. Too, in spiritual life each is given, is confronted with, the precise circumstances and conditions which are most relevant to his needs. Whatever the type of work we are given, it has a meaning. We have to take the work as a chosen field provided for us. Necessarily in endeavours like this there cannot always be regular hours of work. The needs are sudden and the adjustment of rhythm is not so much external as internal. There has to be an inner harmony. One may work at concreting at an unusual time, but the mind can recall and establish contact with that which you are used to doing at that time—be it meditation or study. Even that thought is enough. To remember that it is the time one generally reads *Savitri*, for example, enables the subliminal being to open to the presence presiding over that communion with *Savitri*.

We have necessarily to modify our individual programme to suit the collective's needs. And I have no doubt whatever that in this way and in other ways also, the work for seekers who have gathered here in Auroville is of a different type, and their way and goal is somewhat different than that which was set before the people who came thirty or forty years ago to the Ashram. There is no question of one being easier or more difficult than the other. The type of soul itself is different in each of the two experiments; and there is no question either of one type being more advanced than the other. It is not that. It is that each soul has come for a particular kind of work and experience.

I am deliberately mentioning this because there is a wrong feeling that work and life in the Ashram is preferable to that here. And conversely, in the Ashram there are some people who feel that life in Auroville is freer, easier and preferable. But the truth is that the spiritual life is the same. The way to be trodden depends upon each individual. This particular way is suited for those who are meant to work here, it is not for everybody. Those who have to embody that force of conscious-

ness which is to build the hope of the future are brought
here and given a chance to participate. It is the Divine
who has brought them. If a man rejects that chance and
chooses to go back to the ordinary life, it is his loss. There
is a meaning in people being brought here. It is not by
accident. The Mother has said many times that in her
creation there is nothing left to chance. Everything has
a meaning. She does not allow someone to stay unless
she receives an inner sign. And we have seen that where
we have not left the Mother free to decide these things
but have imposed our preferences, petitions and prayers
in favour of someone, and where she has then yielded,
allowing them to try, things have never worked out suc-
cessfully. Thus after years of observation and experience,
we have now learnt that her first reaction is invariably
correct, and what she says is the best for the individual.
So when she says you are to be in Auroville or else to be
in the Ashram, it means that is the right thing for you.

Which is better, to read aloud or silently?

When the mind is too distracted, when either internally or externally there is distraction, for a few moments to read aloud releases certain physical sound vibrations that create the necessary atmosphere of calm and
peace. But if one is not distracted, the mental vibrations that are released by reading mentally are enough
If one is extrovert by nature, reading aloud helps. But if
one is normally introspective, the Indian shastras considered soundless reading more beneficial. For instance,
in *japa* there are three categories. The lowest is the audi-
ble intonation of the mantra. The second, a little more
advanced, is where only the lips move but no sound is
heard. The third is where there is no physical movement
and no sound, but the repetition of the mantra goes on
inwardly; this is the highest stage. These relate to

different stages of development in the seeker. Certainly when you read aloud a few lines in a book like *Savitri*, they have a great, even therapeutic value. They impregnate the physical atmosphere with a special vibration which has a great spiritual impact even on those around. But for oneself, even a silent reading is enough to feel and to receive those vibrations. In reading aloud, some people lose themselves in the sound, and lose contact with the sense.

9

LOVE IN WORKS

It is possible to consecrate ourselves through knowledge, through the mental sacrifice of acquiring knowledge—learning about the Divine and the divine manifestation—and to put it at the service of the Divine for its extension. It can be a large and wide and pure sacrifice, bereft of the impurities of the lower nature. And for the seeker of the integral ideal, love adds a certain richness and intensity to the quest. The seat of love is the heart; but the heart is suspect to the ratiocinative mind. The mind is always suspicious of the moods, of the undependable fluctuations of the emotions, and it would rather keep the heart out of bounds in the sacrifice of knowledge. But, Sri Aurobindo points out, a strong tradition and spiritual experience testify to the existence of a divine element in the heart which is the fount of all pure emotions and love.

This paradox of the emotive, unpredictable heart being the seat of pure love is resolved when we take into account that actually there is not one heart in man but two, not one soul but two. Most of us are aware only of the surface or outer heart, which is the seat of the desire-soul. The emotive heart and the sensational being together put forward a projection called the soul of desire. The desire-soul attends exclusively to the fulfilment of the demands of the vital being, and the emotional being at the service of the vital. But behind this surface soul there is the deeper soul, what is called the Self in the Upanishads and ancient treatises of India. Deep within there is a spark of divinity, which in most people

is so tiny compared to the rest of the being still in ignorance that the sages have described it as no bigger than
the thumb of a man. The seat of this inner soul is in the
mystic cave of the heart; not in the physical heart, but
behind what is called the cardiac centre. There are veils
upon veils of consciousness that have to be rent before
we come to the luminous cave within—the heart-cave
as it is called—where burns this flame of divinity. From
this psychic element or essence, this soul-spark, all
impulsions for the diviner movements of life issue.

The psychic is also the seat of what is called the
Immanent Divine. The Divine in manifestation has many
poises: it is above the manifestation, above the universe,
we call it the Transcendental Divine; it is spread all
over the universe, in the cosmos, we call it the Universal
Divine; it is also within each form, within each movement, necessarily within each man, we call it the
Immanent Divine. This Immanent Divine has its central
locus in the inner heart of the being. This is the centre,
the real basis for the sacrifice of love to be built upon.
As in the yoga of works, here too there is the usual tendency to demarcate two areas of life: the mundane,
supposed to belong to the ordinary movements of life,
and the religious or the semi-spiritual, which supports,
buttresses and encourages the godward movements
alone. A seeker of God is expected to exclude from himself—at any rate from his alert consciousness—the
mundane activities of life and augment only the area of
religious and godward activities. This is out of the
question for the practitioner of the Integral Yoga. Our
aim is to uplift all of life. It does not admit of life's
demarcation into zones—mundane or supra-mundane,
religious or nonreligious. For our purpose this distinction does not hold; all is Divine, and all shall be imparted

the character of this inspiring Divinity. Nor does the other distinction in society inspired by ethics—what is proper and good, and what is not—properly belong to the spiritual domain. Ethics, after all, is a fine flower of the mental consciousness struggling to eradicate from itself the vestiges of the animal past so that it may grow into the full figure of a life in manhood. Ethics is a self-imposed discipline to help man outgrow his animal past; once he does this and becomes aware of the spiritual dimensions of existence, ethics no longer has any claim to rule or govern his life. Humanism—which passes for spirituality in certain sections of humanity—is only a diminution, at best a recognition, of the sense of the one Divine in the universe at the level of mankind. But that by itself is not enough. Humanism as a result of a spiritual consciousness has spiritual value. But humanism as a goal, as an end in itself, does not carry one very far because ultimately one moves within the circle of ignorance chalked out by present-day humanity.

The yoga of love in works proceeds in three stages. The first is to become aware of the soul, the psychic centre, and to develop it. The psychic in most is just an influence, it is not a being governing the entire personality. The soul's expression is severely affected by the state of the instruments through which it has to act from behind; it is often compared to a king who is governed by the moods of his ministers. The mind, the life, the subtle-physical, and the physical all function as so many veils; or, if they are activated, as so many instruments of the awakened psychic being. They can and do add their own colouring to any psychic influence or guidance that comes. Some of the parts, when unenlightened, can pervert and put to their own use the contribution of the psychic being to the general evolutionary development.

It is the business of the seeker to be sincere to himself, to see how far the intimations of the soul are allowed to come to the front in an undiluted form. The ways of mixture and tainting are devious and unimaginably clever. The vital-mind particularly is a cunning perverter and can be very convincing. It is very tempting, too, to believe that the messages transmitted through the vital-mind are psychic messages. But if one is sincere, one always knows. The psychic has the distinctive qualities of purity, peace, joy (not pleasure), and it brings the feeling of a deep oneness and harmony. To the extent these dynamic values operate in one's life, one can be sure that in that measure the psychic influence has begun to permeate one's life movements.

There is a good deal of misunderstanding regarding the voice of the psychic. Many persons have come to grief by listening to voices that they hear within themselves, believing it is the voice of the soul. There are many imposters of the soul. One has to be absolutely sure before following a voice which claims to be the voice of the soul. In fact, it is safer not to follow a voice allegedly coming from the soul unless it conforms to common sense or is corroborated by the teacher—if one is fortunate to have a living teacher.

As the psychic awakens and its influence extends, one becomes aware of the existence of beauty—in Nature, in men, in forms, in movements. Beauty—to use the celebrated expression of Sri Aurobindo—is restored to its high office of interpretation and expression of the Eternal. When the Eternal manifests in form, it takes the shape of beauty. Where beauty is lacking, there the manifestation in form is not complete. As the psychic develops and casts its influence and light on the outer being, one awakens to the existence of beauty. One also

awakens to the necessity of moulding one's life in this
figure of beauty. Similarly, one awakens to an uncaused
joy, a joy not dependent on any external factor, but a
joy that is a self-existent current of bliss. That joy cir-
culates within and flows out with one's very breath. At
its highest, it uplifts those in one's vicinity. When one is
in that psychic poise, there is an effortless elevation of
all in one's environment. Those who come within such
a person's physical aura, feel a certain warmth, uplift-
ment, and inexplicable purity.

The characteristic power of the psychic being, however, is love. Love is the other face of divine beauty. Just
as consciousness expresses itself in knowledge, force
expresses itself in power and might, the delight of the
Divine formulates itself as love. Love is the link between
God and the world; it is also the link between man and
God. Sri Aurobindo has written in *Eric:* " Love is the
hoop of the gods / Hearts to combine." In this multi-
plicity of creation where forms are divided a millionfold,
they are brought together by the Divine through the
power of love. And love exists between forms on Earth—
between men and animals and plants and matter, between any two units of creation—because the one Divine
indwelling a form calls to the Divine embodied in
another form. "Love", says Sri Aurobindo, "is a yearn-
ing of the One for the One." It is because the Divine in
me is also embodied in you that there is an affinity, that
there is an attraction and interchange in the external
realm. At the purest level it is the One becoming aware
of itself in different stations. But the One undergoes many
changes and variations, and at each level it expresses
itself differently: at the soul level there is a pure love;
at the mental level there is a certain identity of interest,
we call it affinity; at the vital-physical level it may

express itself as passion, as attraction. But whatever the expression, all these movements have at their base the love divine. Human love, with all its perversions and diminutions, is still—or can still be made—a channel, a door to reach the divine love.

Twenty years ago a young seeker in the Ashram asked the Mother whether an aspirant who has taken to the Integral Yoga should eliminate a love that is merely human. Others of us present had only one answer based upon what we had read and understood, and that was that human love is to be excised. We were all flabbergasted when the Mother told him no. She said in effect that one should not cancel human love. Love is to be deepened and enlarged. One must take the best from love and consecrate it, expand it. If one gives oneself entirely, one reaches the border of divine love. Should one deny oneself human love, most likely the heart will dry up and one side of the personality will be denied the Divine manifestation of joy and bliss.

This is certainly not to be taken as a licence, but as with all things in God's creation, human love can be made a definite step towards the borders of divine love. Naturally, human love is not permanent. At best it is a preparation and a starting point for the journey on the path of love. By its very nature, if one is sincere in one's love, one cannot simply remain statically where one is. There has to be a self-giving to another. One learns to eliminate the selfishness and demands that are characteristic of human love. If love is not merely lust or a self-regarding movement masquerading as love, it is a dynamic force. It touches certain depths of the being and awakens and prepares the being for higher intensities of life. All depends upon sincerity. Sri Aurobindo has written:

> Love men, love God. Fear not to love . . .
> From self escape and find in love alone
>   A higher joy.

"From self escape", that is, free yourself from the circle
of your ego. Through love we find our kinship with the
sky. If we learn first to love our family, and then our
neighbours, community, society, and so on, there is an
enlarging circle of love which ultimately reaches the
vastnesses:

> By love we find our kinship with the stars.

Love is

> . . . the sign
> Of one outblaze of godhead that two share.

And,

> To live, to love are signs of infinite things,
> Love is a glory from eternity's spheres.
> Abased, disfigured, mocked by baser mights
> That steal his name and shape and ecstasy,
> He is still the Godhead by which all can change.

How does love grow?

> And Love that was once an animal's desire,
> Then a sweet madness in the rapturous heart,
> An ardent comradeship in the happy mind,
> Becomes a wide spiritual yearning's space.

Love begins on Earth but does not end with Earth. Love
is the bridge between Earth and heaven. Love must not
seek to live only upon Earth forever, yet:

> Love must not cease to live upon the earth;
> For Love is the bright link twixt earth and heaven,
> Love is the far Transcendent's angel here;
> Love is man's lien on the Absolute.

It is this expanding movement of love that is to be cultivated. And no one can truly love unless he forgets

himself. One has to die to oneself before one can be
born in the love divine. Even one single ray of divine
love can alter the whole character of one's life.

This sublimation of human love into divine love is
a crucial test in this aspect of the Integral Yoga. It is a
discipline which has to be worked out in detail. There
are, as I said, enemies at work within ourselves who lie
in ambush waiting for such pure and uplifting and trans-
muting movements to come forth; they twist them, they
pervert them—one cannot be too careful. Further, as
the love for the Divine begins to shape itself, one has
necessarily to adore and offer one's worship of love to the
Divine at all levels. It is not difficult to worship the
transcendent Divine, the Lord who is above everything;
but love for the transcendent Divine is not complete
unless it is shared with all in the universe. The transcendent Divine is manifest in the universe in myriad forms,
and love has to be given to the Divine manifest in the
universe, in man, in every form.

And here we come to the crux of the worship of
God in images. The original idea was, indeed, to perceive
the divine presence in these forms where the divine consciousness has been concentrated by an adept. But at
times, as happens in this world, the outer form has
remained but the inner spirit has departed. The seeker
of the integral path has to keep the formless in mind even
when he worships the form. Looming over the limited
form is the presence of the Eternal, the unnameable, the
undefinable, the formless Divine. When you worship an
image or even a man as a teacher, it is to this Divine that
you offer your adoration. From this point of view, every
movement in life has to be suffused with the spirit of
love. Love not for oneself, not for one's interest, but love
for the one Divine indwelling all.

10

LOVE EXTENDED

In our study of "the ascent of the sacrifice", we have seen that the life of man is a constant ascent—whether he is aware of it or not—from darkness to light, from nonbeing to being, from ignorance to knowledge. The ascent is also the road of sacrifice. And it is a sacrifice not in the sense in which the term is normally understood but in the sense of a self-consecration, a giving up of oneself to the Divine in and above the universe. This cosmic sacrifice has been in progress since the Creator gave birth to the universe. It is in that sacrifice that our life is meaningful or not. Whether or not we are cognisant of it, whether or not it is our will, we are borne in this movement of sacrifice.

A seeker of the Divine analyses the different movements of the sacrifice and discovers its root significance so that he may participate in it consciously. We have seen the part of the yoga of knowledge in the sacrifice. And we have studied the role of love in the sacrifice of life and the truth that is behind love, or rather the truth that is love. Love is the keelson of creation, as the poet put it. It is an original creative force, an irresistible power. Out of love the universe has emerged, and in and through love is its salvation.

We have considered love in its general dimension. Now the theme is how precisely the yoga of works in the ascent of the sacrifice involves the path of love. It may or may not be conceivable to the mind how human love can be transmuted by the alchemy of Grace into a divine, causeless and selfless love. One must have a certain perception of its possibilities. But just how is this perception and experience of love to be expressed, to be worked out in day to day life, and particularly in works, duty, and service?

There are saints and mystics of all traditions who have opened to the rule of love in their soul, rejecting the actions of life and closing themselves in the cloister of the soul. And there they adore the Beloved, perhaps allowing a few currents of love to flow toward the world. They demarcate the activities of life that can promote the movement of love in the heart, and reject all others as irrelevant if not contrary. Those who may be called humanitarians bring in the element of ethics. They say that philanthropic activities which help the progress of humanity, which strengthen its sense of morality and give wider opportunities, are germane to the seeker of divine love.

Sri Aurobindo says that such distinctions and demarcations mean very little to the seeker of the integral ideal. For the aim is to accept the whole world, to irrigate the field of life with streams of love that flow from the heart centre, to enrich every life-activity with the sap of love. The seeker's intent is to turn all of his life into an adoration of the Divine. Some question whether the Divine would care to accept a consecrated offering of the commonest act of day to day life. Sri Aurobindo cites in this connection the famous lines in the Gita where the Lord declares that whether you offer a leaf, a flower, a cup of water, or any thing or act, he accepts it if there is the spirit of devotion behind it. He accepts what man gives. He responds to every approach of man; as man approaches, so the Lord accepts. This being the declaration of the Divine, Sri Aurobindo exalts all activities of life into means for the adoration of the Divine.

He makes a distinction between the form of the act and the spirit of the act. He does not agree with those purists who say that form is inconsequential provided the spirit is right. Sri Aurobindo gives equal importance to both the form and the spirit of an offering. He is one of the few mystics or thinkers who has given full importance to physical form. He records elsewhere, also, that the outer form is the just configuration of the spirit of the consciousness that seeks to express itself.

As the consciousness grows and changes, the subtler eye can perceive changes even in the contours of the physical form. So the precise manner of doing the act is as important as the attitude behind it. Herein lies the truth of physical worship. Intellectuals and monistic spiritualists are inclined to dismiss worship as a mode belonging to the domain of the ignorant. But there is a profound truth expressed in the form of external worship. Living as we do on the physical plane, a physical form of worship has the positive advantage of concretely establishing the consciousness that seeks to organise itself on Earth. Possibly on the higher or subtler planes, forms are constantly changing; whereas on Earth, forms are more firmly fixed. Most of us have through our dreams an insight into this truth. We see in dreams figures changing form; this adaptibility of form belongs to the subtler planes. On the physical plane, each precise form has a meaning. That is why Mother is so particular about perfection in expression, in form. Beauty is the expression of truth on the physical plane.

Thus, each element of worship is significant: the act itself, its symbolic aspect, and the awareness that it represents a movement of consecration, a movement of reaching out to the Divine. There is a moment to moment exertion of seeking for the Divine not only above but also around, in the universe. One must grow conscious that it is the Divine in so many different forms and centres that receives one's offering. Work is done not only with love for the Divine who is seated in one's own heart, but for the Divine in all creation. Love flows to the million-bodied love, to the God of love with myriad souls. That love has a liberating force. It is creative love.

It may be asked: If love has such a creative force as ascribed to it by Sri Aurobindo and the Mother, why is it that we do not see love flourishing on Earth; why is love not a dominating force even after millions of years of evolution? It is not a flourishing or dominating force because of the sense of division, because of the separativity in consciousness. Each individuated unit separates from the rest. Though man has advanced in many ways beyond his ancestors of thousands of years ago, it is very rare that he truly loves others. His sole occupation and preoccupation is to act for his own benefit. He exerts himself in his own interests and for others so long as it subserves his interests. His service to others and his interest in them is commonly motivated by self-interest, overt or disguised. It is only as man grows beyond the belt of ignorance and selfishness that he begins to awake to the need of exerting himself truly for others. It is a matter of evolution, evolution of consciousness. Only when there is a widening of the mind and consciousness can the true vibrations of love in action be felt.

The aim of this yoga is to discover love at one's source. Love is at the source of all but it is most easy to discover it at the source of one's own being. Like a gentle spring it issues forth. Like a current it flows. In our purest moments, when we forget ourselves and the mind is still, love awakes. When the love divine comes for-

ward, there is no excitement. There is felt a silent bliss
that is eternal. The whole universe floats in a sea of love.

To this awakening of the love within and its extension into the corridors of the being there are obstructions at every step. Obstructions from the obscurity of
the physical body, the impurities of the turbid flow of
life, the knots of ego, the crookedness of the cunning
mind and the aridities of the logical mind, all combine
to break up this movement of love. They either fragment it or twist it; they give it a shape that perverts it
totally out of character.

The only way, Sri Aurobindo points out, to prevent
this sort of distortion of the divine love that has begun
its outflow is to awaken the psychic being. At the outset, the psychic being also has the same difficulty. Every
ray of its light, of its influence, is interrupted by the
numerous intervening veils between the surface being
and the psychic at the core. By sheer aspiration and invocation, the psychic being must be strengthened. By
helpful movements of the surface nature, constant remembrance and dwelling upon its need to come forward,
the psychic being has to be drawn out. As it is said in
one of the Upanishads, it is to be drawn out like a thin
fibre from a blade of grass. The psychic is to be brought
forward, strengthened, listened to, obeyed, given a
shape, and provided scope to develop into a personality.
Only when the psychic being comes forward and sheds
its light on the rest of the movements of the being does
the divine love, or the purer love from within, get an
opportunity to organise itself, to flow outward and suffuse
action in one's day to day life—the sacrifice of works—
with its warmth and purity and creative power.

It is also this psychic power which establishes a bridge between the individual human nature and the power of the truth-will, the gnosis above. There too in its descent to the human plane it faces so many obstructions. But if the psychic door is open and the psychic aspiration shoots up, it is possible for the action of the gnosis, the supramental consciousness, to reach down to the individual soul. And when the supramental consciousness touches the love manifest in man, that love acquires its true dynamic character. The most important result is that one perceives the one Divine in all. One begins to love each created thing in the universe with the same intensity and abundance with which you love the One.

Are there any questions?

Are there actually what are called "psychic tears"?

Everyone likes to think that his tears are expressions of the psychic. There are tears of different types. And also, there is truly a distinction between the weeping of the psychic and the tears of the psychic. The psychic weeps when the outer being insists on behaving stupidly without responding to the pressure from within, when one's nature insists on turning its back on the guidance afforded by the psychic. When the soul is ready for a leap but the outer nature refuses to cooperate, the psychic weeps. If a man does not change when such a situation arises, either the soul leaves the body or the major part of it withdraws, leaving only a fragment to continue till the body is shed.

But psychic tears come when one perceives the Divine either as beauty or as bliss. When you are overcome by the marvel of the divine manifestation, the psychic sheds tears of joy. Or when you are moved by seeing the divine purpose suffering due to the crudity and irresponsiveness in those around, there may be psychic tears. These are tears of regret. But psychic tears don't exhaust one. They bring about a great purifying change. I would not merely say that they have an effect, they register a step ahead.

Would you clarify the point regarding the soul withdrawing under certain circumstances, leaving only a portion of itself in the body to continue?

When the soul is undeveloped it is only a fragment, an entity. But with experience it develops into a personality. It is not confined to the body, though its centre is there. If the soul finds that the body is not responsive to its needs and therefore can no longer serve it, but that the body has some karma remaining to be worked out, a fragment of the soul may continue and the major part withdraw. That is why you see some who have been outstandingly spiritual at some stage in their life begin to deteriorate; their inner being withdraws. But it does not force the body to drop away. The embodiment has to work out certain karma. So only the outer shell is left; the real soul has withdrawn. There have been a number of cases where a soul that has come with a certain aspiration has been disappointed and has then chosen to retire, leaving only an outer shell.

An analogy can be seen in dream and out-of-the-body experiences. When the being goes out, a part remains in the body, the whole of the being does not go. Actually what normally happens is that the major part stays in the body and a part of the being is projected elsewhere. But as one develops the occult technique, the central being may go out for its work, work for the Divine or

work of whatever kind, and only a fragment of it continues
to animate the body.

What is the relation of devotion to love?

Even as early as two thousand years ago, Narada
in his famous aphorism on bhakti said that the final
result of devotion is love. Devotion is a general movement, relatively self-regarding. But when the dross of
the personal element of self-interest falls away and devotion turns itself into an absolutely God-regarding movement where one forgets oneself, it becomes adoration.
And this adoration develops into love. Inner devotion,
passing through the stage of adoration, reaches its climax
in love. In the section of *The Synthesis of Yoga* on the way
of love is an exceedingly beautiful description of this
gradation. Love is the fine fruit of devotion.

11

THE CORE OF THE YOGA OF WORKS

Now we shall deal with the yoga of works, proper. Whether it is knowledge or love, ultimately they have to be expressed in dynamic terms on the level of practical life. The yoga of works concerns the actual dynamisation of the will in the life-force. Life is impossible without effort. Where there is life there is movement, activity. It is said in the Gita that no one can live and breathe unless there is some outflow of energy, some activity.

Here we come to the crux of another problem. It has been a traditional attitude to consider work as foreign to genuine spirituality. It is said that work belongs to the field of Nature, and God to the field of the soul; that the two do not meet. They may overlap at certain points on the journey, but they ultimately have to part. That is because the field of work and life-energy is considered to be contaminated. One may start with a pure motive, but one gets bogged down at some stage. That is why works are to be rejected. But if works are inevitable, it is argued, let us do only those works which are indispensable for the maintenance of the body; or, to make a concession, those works which nourish the upward aspiration, second it without involving the higher effort of the soul godward—works like worship, prayer, and adoration. Perhaps one can add works of philanthropy in order to purify oneself, to throw away the dross of selfishness and thus lighten one's burden on the way. Thus in all traditions, Eastern and Western, works are frowned upon as distracting and foreign to the central purpose of the spiritual quest. But the seeker of the integral path cannot afford to subscribe to this view. The very object of this yoga is the elevation of life, the perfection of life, the transformation of life as it is into its higher term.

It is not possible to wait till the way of knowledge has sufficiently enlightened the being for one to safely launch upon the yoga of works. Nor is it possible to wait till the yoga of love has purified and readied the being to begin the sacrifice of works. Because whether it is knowledge or love, they need the support of the life-force. After all the life-force is the link between spirit and matter, between mind and matter, between love and matter. It is the life-force that has to dynamise these eternal and higher values in terms of life. If knowledge is divine in its origin, if love is divine in its origin, even the much abused life-force, Sri Aurobindo says, is absolutely divine in its origin. Life-force is a power of God.

In its original purity it is a projection of the pure force of consciousness at the head of manifestation. Just as the supramental consciousness projects itself as the mental consciousness in the lower triple world, just as the pure existence congeals itself as solid matter, and just as the infinite bliss formulates itself as the psychic principle, the consciousness-force—chit-shakti as it is called in Indian terminology—projects itself as the life-force. In its native character, power—which is the characteristic of life-force—is neither good nor bad, moral nor immoral. It depends upon what use it is put to. If the works of the life-force in the day to day life of the world have a tendency to involve man in the petty rounds of egoism and lower nature, it is because—through the general deformation that has come over the world in the course of involution and evolution—the life-force is controlled by and made subservient to the desire-soul. In the course of evolution, desire, which is a first motive for action in this world of ignorance, has by sheer habit formed a centre of reference that is the desire-soul. No action is undertaken without some impelling desire-motive. The desire-soul is the root of this deformation of the original creative and liberative life-force into a force for bondage.

Once he is engaged in the yoga of works, the first step for the seeker of the integral path is to become conscious of this element in him: the desire-soul which has to be rejected. It is not easy to reject such a formidable and ages-old formation in the nature. It is enough as a first step that one is sincere and discriminating enough to feel and scrutinise where desire comes into play. A ruthless analysis of oneself is called for. This is indispensable if the desire-soul's hold over the nature is to be weakened. Once one goes to the root of this problem and isolates the desire-soul, the true being of the life-force, the true vital being begins to emerge. And this inner vital being is a warrior of the Divine. It is the agent of the divine consciousness projected in evolution at the life level. It is its effectuating agent. And when this inner vital being is gradually induced to come out and assume charge, one feels a flood of energy, a mighty wave of power, and a limitless capacity virtually takes possession of one's being. It is not easy to support this rush of the inner vital being. It is very easy for the lower elements of the nature to infest this emergent vital being, the true being of life-force, and deflect its purpose. That is why Sri Aurobindo and the Mother insist upon merciless purification of motive—an inner cleanliness with no allowance for subterfuge, no toleration of the cunning of the vital mind. To this end it is necessary to invoke the psychic being which is behind the surface personality, behind the desire-soul.

After all, what we call the human personality, what passes for the soul, is the desire-soul, the ego formation. It is only a shadow of the inner soul. And the inner soul as projected in evolution is the psychic being, the delegate of the immanent Divine in evolution. This psychic presence or being is to be enlivened and induced to come forward and preside over the activity of the emergent vital being. Left to itself the vital being does not have the necessary sense of direction or the illumination. It acts and effectuates where it is directed to do so. Guidance of the psychic being is necessary. By devotion, by purification, eliminating all contrary movements, by aspiration, by the cultivation of the elements of beauty, love, harmony, and peace, not creates the climate for the psychic influence to slowly organise the ground for the psychic being to come to the front and take charge.

But the psychic guidance and control is not the supreme guidance, wisdom or control. The psychic is more or less a light to show the way, to point out which is the right and which the wrong way. It is a witness consciousness acting when it is waited upon. It is not a self-sufficient power which is capable of guiding man to an ultimate goal. It is a helper on the way. The psychic is a delegate of the parent Divine, and it summons to the situation a divine power. Above the triple nature of mind, life, and body, there is waiting a divine presence, the divine shakti, which is even now guiding from behind the veil. Once the psychic is brought to the front and the aspiration joined to it, the next step is to invoke this higher power beyond the realm of the triple nature to guide.

This is what Sri Aurobindo calls the intervention of the consciousness-force of the Divine. But this divine shakti does not precipitate matters or manifest itself immediately because the human receptacle is not yet ready. If the divine puissance were to manifest itself at a stroke, the unprepared being would be dashed to pieces like an unbaked vessel under pressure. Unless it is prepared and readied by the fire of *tapasya*, askesis, the human body is sure to crack under the direct impact of the mighty puissance. That is why the Divine in its providence intervenes gradually. It acts and then withdraws till the nature assimilates the working of the higher power; it then waits till the being is ready for another intervention.

These alternating periods are referred to as day and night by the Vedic mystics. The days are the bright periods when all is handled by a higher force; all is joyous, bright, and sweetened by the current of love and harmony emanating from the psychic being. It is a time of wonderful, smooth progress. But it cannot last. Nature demands time to assimilate. The lower elements—the demands of the physical body, the habits of the vital, the grooves of the mental being—insist on following their old ways, and they pull one down. Then the higher power withdraws till the gains made are assimilated, organised, and made part of the being. These are the nights of the soul, what is called elsewhere the sloughs of despond. But in the Veda, they are simply called nights, the times of relative or actual darkness which follow the luminous times of day.

It is by a constant invocation, reception, and utilisation of higher descents of the power, guided at our level by psychic perception, that this journey of the sacrifice in works towards God proceeds. These are the three

steps: elimination of the desire-soul; letting the true
vital being come forward under the guidance of the
psychic being; evocation of the higher power, the
divine shakti, to accept the sacrifice and, in time, to
even conduct the sacrifice.

Translated in other terms, it means that one has in
day to day life to give up desires for the fruits of work.
Of course it is not possible to give up desire immediately
and entirely. But in the beginning, at least in the main
work that one does, one shall not think of the fruits of
the work. One does the work that is allotted, that is
given by circumstances, or that falls to one's share. And
one does it to the best of one's ability as a dedication,
self-consecration, but one does not desire a particular
fruit. Once this desire for the fruit is abandoned, the
next element to be rejected is the desire for a particular
work. There should be no personal choice or preference.
Whatever work comes has to be done in an impersonal
manner. And the true evidence indicating whether or
not one has given up desire is the presence of equality.
Do I react to situations, to men, and to things with equality? Does success elate me? Does failure depress me?
If I come across difficult situations, am I disturbed?
Do I feel upset or downgraded if my view does not
prevail? If I don't possess equality it means that I am
still in the grip of desire. And behind desire is ego.

This is the first practical step that a seeker has
to take. Second, to become conscious of the psychic
presence and shape one's life so that the rays of the
psychic emerge in the front. Third, to open oneself to
the higher regions of the mind and the widenesses of the
heart so that the transcendent power of the Divine finds
a receptive opening for its descent, ingression, and extension. These are capital steps in the yoga of works. And

there are three stages in the sacrifice of works: first, one gives up the fruit of work to the Divine; second, one leaves the choice of work to the Divine; third, one loses the sense of the doer of work. One becomes first an instrument; then one loses even the sense of being an instrument, one becomes just an unresisting channel of the divine force; finally, one is simply identified with the divine shakti and becomes one with it.

Does anyone have any questions?

Is the worker expected to take joy in whatever work he is asked to do?

Certainly. It is legitimate and expected that the worker experiences the delight of work. Ultimately the meaning of all life is delight. There is a divine delight that underflows all movements. And the truer the spirit in which one works, the greater the felicity which flows into the being. One should take the joy of work, communicate it if possible, but one shall not be attached to that work. If the work is changed, one should be able to link oneself with that same stream of joy. It is not the work that is important. It is the spirit of consecration and the way in which one works out the consecration that is important. It is that that gives joy. It is when one is linked with the Divine through the channel of work that the delight flows. That should happen whatever the work one does. One should certainly enjoy what one does, but in the true spirit. All life is a flow of bliss, and it is a sign of one's touching the depths of life when one effortlessly feels this course of bliss. If one feels a certain joy in work here for the Divine that one could not have derived in similar work elsewhere, it only shows that the work here is organised on a different level and that

one does it on a deeper level than one could have elsewhere. One is helped to do it in the right spirit and at
the right level. The results are evident; but they are left
in the hands of God. Ours is but to work.

How can we feel and recognise the psychic guidance?

It is to be felt and recognised within. But it is not
easy to recognise the psychic presence or influence. It is
very tricky because the emotional being many times
masquerades as the psychic. For instance, the first term
of expression of the psychic is love. But on a human level
the emotional being may feel a certain attraction and
translate it as love. It is very easy to confuse this love of
the emotional being with psychic love. But a true characteristic of psychic love is peace; there is no agitation
or excitement. When the love is emotional, there is
excitement. Psychic love is a quiet, uncaused, self-existent sweetness. This love is a force of harmony, a universal sympathy, an attraction to all that is beautiful. The
psychic has an aversion to ugliness, gossip, and petty
criticism. If someone or something has a defect, it is
compassion that flows, not the working of the critical
faculty.

There is a constant flow of the inner being toward
merging itself with the Divine. Everything reminds one
of the Divine. Life becomes a poem of celestial bliss. But
at times, if one's nature is recalcitrant and obstructive,
there is a psychic sadness, a regret. It may express itself in the form of tears or it may not. But one feels that
the being is not keeping pace with the soul.

The psychic guidance carries with it a certain
conviction. One knows that it is true. Its indications of
what is right and what is wrong are self-evidently valid.

One does not have to ponder over the guidance, one feels convinced that it is true.

There is an effortless perception wherever one looks of the nature of a thing. The ego's posturing is absent, and one feels soiled or tainted at the first return of selfishness. One feels terribly impure at any surge of passion or anger. These are signs of the presence of the emergence of the psychic.

What do you mean when you say that the psychic is unhappy?

Essentially the psychic cannot be unhappy, but the evolving psychic being, because of its participation in the outer nature's thoughts and feelings, can feel denied or constrained when the nature refuses to cooperate. Psychic sadness is its reaction expressed in our surface nature. Even if one sees no apparent reason why one should be sad, one sometimes is. This may be caused, for instance, when one leaves the Ashram, even if only for a brief while. It is not that there is a lower attachment, it is that the soul feels unhappy at being physically away from its Mother Soul. There is regret. I suppose evolution in human terms implies these side effects.

Is the psychic present in all? How does it act?

In most, the psychic is present merely as an essence. In the course of evolution this psychic essence develops into an entity. The psychic entity does not yet have a personality. But when experience after experience is gained by that entity on higher and higher grades of consciousness, it develops into a being. And when the psychic being develops into a personality, man reaches the stage when he enters spiritual life. No one enters true spiritual life unless the development of his psychic has arrived at the stage of the development of the psychic being.

This psychic being does not come forward immediately. It first exerts its influence through an indirect touch. When as a result of this constant influence, the nature is ready, it sends a direct emanation. The emanation may be imaged as a ray, a projection of its consciousness. It is something more than an influence. And when by the constant working of this psychic emanation the nature is fully ready, the psychic being itself comes to the front and dominates and leads the triple formation of the mental being, the life being, and the physical being. Till then, the psychic being holds them from behind. When it emerges, it assumes control over all three.

This is more or less the course of development of the psychic being: it begins as the Divine's spark, the psychic essence; then assumes form as the psychic entity; and thereafter it develops into a psychic being with a personality of its own, which ultimately rules the whole being.

Do you mean by what you said earlier that one has to always stay in the Ashram for the psychic efflorescence?

No, it is not the case. Even the psychic sadness which I said one feels at physical separation is not a permanent affair. It is only for some time that one feels it. Thereafter, the link is reestablished and one feels in tune, in communion. It is just when one leaves that there is that feeling—for some, not for all. Some don't feel it because they live in constant communion and they carry the link within. But some find it difficult.

This is only an illustration of an instance when the phenomenon of psychic sadness may be felt. Being in contact with the Mother or the Divine as expressed in her, is certainly not determined by physical distance. For those who are in communion with her inwardly, the outer circumstances do not matter. Her presence is felt wherever one is. But those who are not yet developed enough or strong enough to establish that inner link and live in that relation with her, need a preparatory period of living near the central fire so that the being may be prepared. Ultimately, in spiritual matters, physical distance has no relevance. But till the spiritual development has matured to a certain stage, it is incumbent upon some to come close to the source of inspiration and imbibe it. It is not so for all. Those who need it or are called are brought here.

12

STANDARDS OF CONDUCT AND SPIRITUAL FREEDOM

The next area of study concerns standards or norms of behaviour from the point of view of a spiritual seeker. As is today commonly admitted, the time is past when one standard of conduct or one set of standards is expected to be applicable to all. Though throughout history each ruler has wanted to impose the standards of his people on all those whom he conquered. Many were actually very earnest in their belief that their standards of conduct were the ultimate, that they would be good for all. There is a legend, perhaps apocryphal, that when the caliph of Turkey conquered Alexandria in one of his military excursions, he ordered the magnificent library of Alexandria to be burnt down. When he was asked why he had burned such a treasure of wisdom, he said that those books in the library that were contrary to the dictates of the Koran were dangerous and therefore should be burnt. And those which conformed to the Koran were redundant. In either case, they should be burnt. This is typical of the narrow human mentality which considers the standards it practises the ultimate ones.

In India it has always been recognised that standards vary with the competence of the people concerned. In Indian society, there are clearly marked demarcations of competence. This is called dharma. Dharma is not a religion or a code of conduct, it is action according to the ruling law of self-being. At each stage in man's life there is a particular law of operation. His conduct must correspond to that law which is appropriate.

Accordingly, Indian seers devised a system consisting of four stages in the life of man: celibate student; house-holder; mature elder retired from active life; and recluse. There were severe standards for the celibate student which were relaxed only when he reached an age when he could marry and lead a responsible life as a member of the society. More responsibilities were added at the time of his retirement from active life. Once he had fulfilled his obligations to his family and to society and chose to walk into the wilderness of the free Spirit, he was absolved from observing any standards. To this, certain questions are commonly and very naturally asked: "Does this mean that a recluse, a spiritual seeker who has chosen to go beyond the rules of society, can do as he likes? Can he give up the laws of morality? Isn't that an encouragement of immorality in the name of religion and spirituality?" These are very legitimate questions, but considered in the proper perspective, they lose their basis. Standards correspond to the stage of evolution reached by an individual.

There is in the universe a great creative force of evolution, a divine force in action. And every individual action, whether or not one is conscious of it, is a part of the general movement, the universal action. And as man becomes conscious of his part in this universal activity, his attitude to men and things changes. In the beginning when he is largely unconscious of the fact that he is but a fragment of the universal, he is ruled by the needs—or what he fancies to be the needs—and desires of the physical body and vital energy. All rules and norms are erected to subserve his primary needs. At this age, man is primarily a physical man. As are his needs and desires, so are his standards of conduct. In most early societies, such norms are common.

But very soon man finds that he does not live alone; he is a member of a collectivity. This collectivity is first his family, then his clan, then his society. He draws from each collectivity, and each expects and forces him to serve it. Where his individual standards for self-effectuation and self-aggrandisement clash with similar standards erected by other individuals, there is friction. There must therefore be compromise; and thus social law comes into operation. The social standards that thus emerge aim first to control the predatory instincts of the human animal and to ensure that individual interests are accommodated within the collective interests. These interests are harmonised as far as possible, but there is an ever insistent conflict between the individual and the society. The individual claims that the society is a field for his development; and in this he is not wrong. He draws upon the collective wealth around him; he exploits the potentials in the realms of mind, life, and matter around him; and he wishes to be a monarch of all around him. However, Nature counters this claim and effort of the individual with the claim of the society on him. After all, as it is said, the individual is but a cell in the corporate body. And a cell cannot exist except as a part of the larger being; it feeds upon it. If the individual is to survive and progress, it is indispensable that he subordinates himself to and participates in the common progress. Nature experiments with this friction on both sides and tries to strike a balance between the needs of the individual and the claims of the society. That is where the standards of each first comes into conflict. A compromise is worked out. But, as Sri Aurobindo points out, a compromise is hardly a solution; it only complicates matters in the end.

And a third stage arrives when the perception dawns that the true law of conduct is determined neither by one's own physical or vital interests nor the dominating interest of the community. A new ideal is sought which justly accounts for both interests, and something more; thus ethics evolves. Man conceives of a law of God which should control and rule his conduct. Different seers and thinkers conceive of it differently. However, each society erects its own mode of ethics, its own ideal of perfection, and tries to put it into practice. But indeed the lag between practice and precept is wide. Still, the very fact that an effort is being made, at least in the advanced sections of the society, to practise an ideal and to follow the injunctions of ethics, is an indication that man has advanced beyond the elementary stages and has emerged into the domain of mind. It is no longer merely the body and the life-force that dominate man's existence, it is now the enlightened mind that has begun to claim man.

But here too, man experiences conflict between the various ideals that are erected at different times and in different climes. Some conceive the ruling ideal to be justice; some hold it to be knowledge; some consider it to be love. Between these there is conflict. For instance, justice may demand what love abhors; while love may call for something which justice would not allow. This continual conflict in the awakened conscience of man between the various erected ideals convinces him after a time that they are not the ultimate.

There are stages in the life of man and in the growth of the society when mental laws have to be enforced, when rules of morality have to be observed. But it should be recognised that they are not the self-sufficient or ultimate guides for human existence. In India this great error has been made by some leaders who have raised

an ethical ideal to an absolute standard. They have not
hesitated to sacrifice the interests of millions of people
at the altar of such an ideal which is wrongly considered
a universal law. Nonviolence is one such idea. Whether
or not nonviolence is a practical ideal for humanity at
its present stage of development is problematic. Actually,
nonviolence is a law of a plane other than the physical.
Advanced thinkers have begun to perceive that such
ideals are, after all, manmade, mind-made. As the mind
develops, the limitations of these ethical ideals are felt
acutely. But it is a rule of spiritual life that one cannot
forsake an ideal which has governed one's life until one
is ready to follow a higher ideal.

Here I am reminded of an incident which happened
several years ago. There were some rather boisterous
young men here from Europe whom I befriended by
arranging accommodations in one of our guest houses.
After they were given a place to stay, they simply went
wild. They stole things wherever they went and generally
behaved outrageously. When someone spoke to them of
the Ashram discipline and of the need to observe a certain decorum, they said that they did not believe in rules
or discipline and were out to break such "formations".
And they refused to leave after the period for which I
had permitted them was over. So I had to speak to
Mother about the situation. After I told her what was
happening she took out a paper and wrote something for
me to give to them. It said: "You have no right to break
a law unless and until you are ready for a higher law."
I sent it to the man who was the leader of the group. I
was told that when he saw Mother's message, his face
beamed. They left the next day.

I mention this to illustrate that it is not enough just
to say that old standards have no relevance to the new

age. For, they have no relevance only if one has crossed over into another state of consciousness or being beyond the range of application of earlier laws or ideals. And the Mother has said countless times that it is also not right to disturb the faith of a person, however unenlightened he may appear, unless one can replace it by a greater and deeper faith. Till one has such a capacity, one must not interfere.

So these laws and standards of ethics and morality have a part to play in the evolutionary development of man as long as his animal-nature has not been left behind. As long as he continues to be ruled by his ego and desires, these checks are necessary; largely to guard him from his own errors. When a man is ready, when he has realised all that ethics can contribute to his development, and when manmade rules and conventions clearly obstruct his mental and spiritual progress, only then is it the time to leave aside these standards and look to others which are a higher self-formulation of the divine law of truth.

The divine truth formulates itself into the verities of love, knowledge, and compassion. And when man arrives at their level, they function harmoniously, without conflict, and help him to radiate their common truth in the society.

Though individuals may arrive at this spiritual level of consciousness, the whole of society is obviously not at that stage or ready for it. The individual always leads and holds the key of progress. This is true even in the spiritual realm. The enlightened individual has to be the torchbearer of the gnostic consciousness. As individuals who govern themselves by standards of spiritual conduct multiply, and as some degree of cohesion and solidarity emerges by their common living, their collective soul is formed in the mould of the spiritual consciousness.

Spiritual truth as expressed as a spiritual standard of conduct formulates itself differently for different individuals and in different instances. Though fundamentally it is uniform, it differs in its application. In this there is a great difference between spiritual law and ethical law. Ethical law insists on being applied identically in all cases. But spiritual law applies itself uniquely in each case depending upon the need of the situation, the level of the person's consciousness, and the nature of his call. Thus the spiritual man is catholic, plastic and flexible in his approach to standards of conduct.

These divine standards of conduct are self-effective and self-evident. One does not need to be told what the standards are; one acts spontaneously in their terms. It is a problematic question whether or not humanity has yet arrived at the stage when the rule of conduct according to higher standards can become natural. Prophets have spoken and poets have sung of the kingdom of God on Earth, of the golden age, of the age of truth. If now is to be that time really depends upon the number of and the quality of individuals who first realise this state of consciousness in their own life. As long as men continue to be circumscribed by their personal viewpoint and ruled by their ego, and as long as men do not have the sense of universality and unity with others, all talk of spiritual standards, of the gnostic consciousness, and of supramental way of living, is academic.

Let us then start with what is possible for us at this stage of our evolutionary development. Let us cease to be separate individuals at least in our consciousness and in our way of thinking and feeling. All of us know mentally that we are one at a certain level. There is a divine consciousness and being where we are one, from which we derive. Let each one of us make it a habit at a certain time every day to retire into our depths and from there feel our unity with all, to universalise ourselves in our thoughts and feelings. This identification is done first by imagination, then by thought, then by feelings. It will ultimately develop into an actual fact of life. One embraces the whole Earth and universe with one's love and consciousness. This would be a grand and fit beginning.

Questions?

Was it only after one had passed through the first three stages of life that a spiritual life was possible in Indian society?

The four stages of life in Indian society were only a practical, generally applicable, division. But those individuals who were awakened and felt the call of the Spirit were not obliged to pass through all the three earlier stages. They could withdraw from society and pursue their quest at any time. Too, each of the stages had its own discipline to see that spiritual energies were rightly channelled and that there was no possibility of self-deception and regression.

There were relevant, spiritually based guidelines for each of the preliminary stages. But once the seeker had arrived at a certain fulfilment, he was bound by nothing. He would be what is termed in Sanskrit a *parivrajak;* the nearest English translation of which—though it is not very accurate—is, a recluse. He was not a member of society; he insisted on and was granted his own unfettered way of life.

But if such individuals are not bound by the conventions and morality of society, can they not easily do
anything they want in the name of God? The fact is that
when a man has arrived at a state of consciousness which
places him in a category above the rule of these standards, it is unthinkable that he could have the impulse
to indulge in unethical practices. A man who has attained
to a supra-ethical state normally cannot slide back to
the infra-ethical. A supra-ethical man is never immoral,
though he may be amoral. And he is indifferent to common notions of morality. Another person unable to
resist a temptation is not disqualified in the eyes of the
supra-ethical man from receiving his compassion and
grace. He does not condemn another because he is not
ethical; but a strictly ethical man will condemn him a
hundred times. The heart of a supra-ethical man goes
out in compassion to those who are in distress.

Almost all the religions of the world have today
ceased to be of utility to the spiritual seeker because as
they are practised they are loaded heavily with this
ethical content. This was perhaps all right at the time
and in the conditions in which they were promulgated.
But times have changed; humanity has progressed. The
deterrent of punishment in heaven is no longer relevant.
That stage is finished. The age of those religions is over;
the age of all-ruling ethics is over.

There is an emerging divine power in action throughout the whole universe. Different centres and individuals
perceive it and conceive of it differently. And each one
expresses it in the measure of his understanding and in
a manner governed by his environmental conditions.
But all expressions refer to the phenomenon of an emerging consciousness. The nature of that consciousness as
it has been understood and formulated in other systems

is not precisely that of which Sri Aurobindo speaks. What some other thinkers speak of is a transcription in their mental consciousness of what is going on behind the scenes. Sri Aurobindo explained long ago that when truths are trying to manifest, they find expression wherever there is some opening, at any level. So the expressions naturally differ depending upon the level of perception and the mould of the receiving mind. It is also possible that the same truths can be expressed identically in two different places. It is the same truth everywhere that is pressing for expression. And for that truth there is no time or space. But the perception of others of the content of that new consciousness is different from the vision of the truth-consciousness of Mother and Sri Aurobindo. Most other conceptions speak in terms of the perfection of humanity at its highest level within the present boundaries. They do not regard humanity as a step toward another level of consciousness, the supramental. And an intermediate race has first to come, form itself, and prepare the ground before a supramental race can project itself on Earth. There is still a big gap between the highest levels of humanity today and the supramental being to come.

What do you mean when you say that the supramental race will "project itself on Earth"?

All formations are not present on the physical plane. There are so many planes where formations are constantly gathering before they precipitate themselves on the physical plane. Many forms are still being worked out on the subtler planes. And it is very likely that the supramental being may appear in that way. If the example of past evolution is to be believed and repeated, the supramental being will be a precipitation.

So too, the first man to appear on Earth was not a direct product of evolution. The evolution of the man-like ape reached a stage where further evolution was not then possible. It was at that point that the creative Divine projected the human type from a subtler plane. And thereafter the possibility was established for man to emerge. Because the first man was a precipitation and not a direct evolute, scientists speak of a missing link in evolution. The missing link does exist, but it is there above, not here. Similarly, as I conceive it and as I have reason to believe, the first supramental man will be precipitated on Earth by an "occult" process of which Sri Aurobindo has spoken in *The Supramental Manifestation upon Earth*. But that manifestation presupposes certain conditions on Earth. The degree of evolution of the ape had brought things to a climactic point where Nature could assimilate and support a higher species. Similarly, a solid ground must be prepared in the consciousness of humanity which will support the spiritual charge and the manifestation of the supramental man. And that is precisely the role of institutions like the Ashram and Auroville: to prepare a favourable, a receptive ground for the higher manifestation to take place.

13

TOWARDS THE SUPREME WILL

We were speaking last time of standards of conduct and the attitude of a spiritual seeker towards them. We noted that these standards are erected by the mind of man to meet certain needs which arise in the course of the evolution of humanity. We concluded that each set of standards is relevant to the particular stage of development to which it answers. Once man passes on to another stage, the old standard ceases to apply and it is replaced by a new one. This being the truth of such standards, it is indispensable that the attitude of an awakened man towards them be flexible. He must adjust as far as he himself is concerned, and be understanding as far as others are concerned.

In the course of the evolutionary journey of the soul there are, Sri Aurobindo points out, three main stages. First, the stage of physical life which is governed mostly by needs and desires. Here, standards are evolved in order to help man to exploit his environment and to build up his life in terms of these two truths—desire and need—of that stage of life. Standards serve to regulate his needs and desires when they come into conflict with the needs and desires of others. The standards, which are at first individualistic, gradually become elastic and expand so as to contain the needs and requirements of others. For the seeker at this stage there is a growing realisation as he develops that this is after all only a very preliminary stage. Once he aspires for the spiritual life, he decides that his own physical comfort and his vital or emotional desires can no longer be the rule. He surrenders these claims of his nature to God. That,

however, is a central decision. It has to be worked out;
the whole of life has to be organised according to this
central directive. But because of the impetus of past
associations, past karmic influences, one's nature often
takes its own course whatever may be the decision of the
enlightened part of the being. But in this there is a purpose. First, to exhaust the karma that has been forged.
Second, to convince the vital part of man from which
desire proceeds that even when this desire is fulfilled it
does not bring the expected satisfaction or contentment.
The same desire fulfilled in the life of a nonseeker has
a different effect. But in the life of a seeker or sadhak,
there is no elation, no lasting joy. One suddenly feels
empty. One feels it was not worth the energy and time
spent in the satisfaction of the desire. One feels it would
have been better to eliminate it at the very outset. Till
this feeling of the vanity of desire and the insufficiency
of a desire-life dawns on man, the lower movement, the
first stage, is bound to persist. Gradually, however, the
pull of the lower desires and needs of life fades, and an
inner orientation, an upward pull, asserts itself.

Once man has arrived at a sufficient expression of
his impulse for personal aggrandisement on the level of
desire, there comes the next, the second stage. There is
an enlargement of his life, an extension of his ego. That
is the beginning of an emotional, social, and mental life
in which he experiences an engulfing contact with his
environment. It is the beginning of the rule of emotions,
ideas, and certain psychic influences. The standards of
conduct at this stage of human development are wider;
they reflect something of the realms of the mind and of
idealism.

But this too is not the end. After a certain stage man
does discover that even this larger edition of himself

becomes a closed book unless the psychic too advances. Society as a whole does not advance beyond the point of the average man. It is the responsibility of the leaders of thought in society to pull it upwards to the third level. There the compulsive hold of mental ideals gives room to the more flexible and mobile standards of the soul.

The highest that the social standard of morality and ethics can evolve is to what Sri Aurobindo calls the *sattvic* ideal, the full man. But to arrive at full manhood in terms of sattvic virtue is not the goal. Sri Aurobindo says elsewhere that the golden chain is to be broken no less than the leaden fetters. The manmade chain of self-satisfying and self-complacent virtue has to be broken. And virtue is a relative term. Where there is virtue there is vice. Where there is neither vice nor virtue, the real truth reigns. So, Sri Aurobindo points out, the next advance is from manhood towards soulhood. For after all, the soul is greater than man. It is when the advanced section of thinking and aspiring humanity arrives at this stage of articulate soulhood that the deeper impulsions of the psychic being, the higher influences of the spiritual reality, begin to assert themselves. A stage arrives when all manmade standards are relegated to the background and each individual has his own standard relevant to his stage of development. Side by side with the emergence of this standardless stage—standardless in the sense of the absence of a universally applicable standard—there is the natural development of understanding and tolerance towards the standards of others which may be at variance with one's own. What is relevant and right for the development of another may not hold good for me; but on that account his standards are not less true. They are true for him. All standards are, in the eyes of the awakened seeker, true to those for whom they are meant.

With this catholic outlook, the whole meaning of standards changes. Standards are regulating guides for the control, elimination, and transcendence of the ego. And what after all is the ego? Man is apt to think that he is the doer, the chooser, the sanctioner, that he is at the root of all action around him. Analysed properly, we find that this " I " which is so loud and prominent, and around which we seek to organise our lives, is neither here nor there. If we look closely within ourselves to discover where the " I " is, we find that this formation simply disappears. But there is an immutable, uninvolved, regarding witness; there is a witness soul. If we go still deeper, the witness yields to the one who sanctions activity. Deeper yet, there is the one who presides over action. Either way, it is not the " I " we are accustomed to, but it is something else. It is the soul, the inner being in its various poises of witness, sanctioner, and presiding power.

Or we may look at the surface being. What is it that effectuates and achieves? It is an energy, a power; it is nature. It is a vast energy of nature channeled into an individual mould. It is a universal force that flows into a channel and effectuates itself through it. So outside it is nature-force, inside it is soul-force. But where is the " I "? The " I " is nowhere. It is a fiction. The ego, the " I " sense, is a fiction erected by evolving nature as a point of centralisation in the flux of life. At each level of our existence, as long as centralisation has not proceeded far enough, it is this ego-point, the psuedo-self, the shadow of the self, that is being strengthened and organised. The physical body functions as a centre for the reception of the outpouring universal physical energy. Our life, the ego of the life-force, is the focusing point of the life energies that flow from all sides. Similarly, the ego in the mind is a point of reference and intersection for the various thought movements, ideas, and idea-forces that continuously criss-cross the mental tier.

Without this ego-point, things would be in a con-tinuous flux. So, it is a strategy of nature to build up this ego entity until the evolving being has arrived at a sufficient power of self-existence and self-development. Once the point of self-possession and self-existence as a separate entity is reached, the purpose and function of the ego is over. The shadow has to give place to the real form which it pretends to be. The soul, the Self, has to come forward. It is the will of the soul, of the being with-in, that must replace the preference, the pseudo choice, and the volition of the outer ego.

In this process man becomes aware of two powers in himself. First, the outer executive nature, called Prakriti in Indian philosophy and, related to it, the soul-power within which is called the Purusha—Prakriti and Purusha, nature and soul. As they function in this world of ignorance, these are in their dynamic move-ment two separate powers. They are separate from each other. The nature-power works, executes; the soul regards. And in its very regard, there is the sanction for the work of nature. The sanction is itself a participation. And this participation reveals itself at a still deeper level as the presiding influence over the activity of nature. This realisation of the relation of Purusha and Prakriti, soul and nature, in oneself, is the first step. It is not the only one. In order to realise this double poise of Purusha and Prakriti, it is first necessary that one detaches oneself from all activity. It is only when one disinvolves oneself from this preoccupation with nature-activity, when one stands back and watches what is

going on—in some part of the being at least—that one
begins to experience freedom from nature. With detachment comes the witness poise. Thereafter, it is a matter
of fulfilling a process till one becomes fully aware of the
Purusha, of the soul in oneself.

Behind this double truth of Purusha and Prakriti
is a more conscious manifestation of the divine, biune
reality. There is a more fully awakened presiding Soul,
the Ishwara, and an equally conscient, impartable
power of that God, the Shakti. The difference between
Purusha and Prakriti and Ishwara and Shakti is this:
Purusha and Prakriti are two separate powers who in
their interaction keep the universal movement going;
Ishwara and Shakti are not two separate powers, Shakti
belongs to Ishwara and embodies the will of Ishwara.
The Shakti functions because of the presence of Ishwara
that she carries. Ishwara himself is not separate from the
Shakti; it is his own power and projection, the projection of his will backed by his vision, that is the Shakti.
They are one reality bifurcated into two, or actually,
poised in two statuses for the purpose of manifestation.

Thus, after the realisation of the Purusha and the
Prakriti comes the deeper and more fulfilling realisation
of Ishwara and Shakti. Mark that this means that in
each one of us there is a double reality, whether one is
a man or woman. Both the poise of the creator, the
conscient soul, and of the dynamic power are embodied
in each individual. The supreme will above projects
itself into the manifestation in this double poise. As one
goes through the stages of detachment, observation, and
realisation of the reality of the Purusha and Prakriti,
one enters into the truth of the dynamic relation between Ishwara and Shakti. At this stage of realisation,

the puny will, the power of choice exercised by the ego, is dead and gone. It is the higher and supreme will alone that is now real.

Naturally, this replacement of the individual will by the supreme will is not attained in a day. It comes in the course of sadhana in three well-marked stages. The first is when one is open and there are moments when the individual will is in tune with the supreme will and functions as its channel. It is an intermittent operation, not continuous. The second stage is when the period of possession of the individual will by the Supreme is extended more and more. That will works through intuition in the heart and direct or indirect command till this periodical possession or guidance yields to the third stage, a gradual fusion and identity with the supreme will.

Questions?

How to rise above Prakriti?

If one develops the habit of carefully observing what one does in the routine of day to day life, one finds many movements which do not faithfully reflect one's higher aspiration, one's central will for consecration. These movements which take place in spite of one's will to the contrary, are the movements of nature, Prakriti. Along with this observation and recognition, there must be the process of isolation of those lower or inferior activities. With this constant observation accompanied by detachment from, and suppression and rejection of, the lower movement, one becomes conscious of a certain purification of the movements of the Prakriti in keeping with the developing aspiration of the Purusha. A part of the mind should always be detached from what one is doing and engaged in observing—pointing out errors and pitfalls, and the wrong appearances which the mind gives to what one is doing.

This observation and analysis of one's self and movements—which necessitates a mental self-honesty—is the first stage of becoming aware of the play of Purusha and Prakriti in oneself. One has to systematically shift one's centre of consciousness from Prakriti, outer nature, inwards towards the soul. Once one does it sincerely and persistently, it develops into a positive habit. Then even in moments in which one is normally unconscious, that habit asserts itself. Whether one yields to the movement of nature or not, one is conscious at that time that it is a foreign movement.

So what is first required, as the Mother says, is sincerity. Once one has chosen the spiritual life, the light of sincerity must be thrown on all that one does and think and feels. Sincerity grows. If one then allows dissimulation and insincerity to rule, it is spiritual suicide. Evolving Nature helps all who want to be free from the clutches of the outer, lower nature. The higher Nature is pressing upon man to grow. From below the soul is aspiring. One has only to be sincere and throw one's weight in the right direction. After a time there need not even be a struggle. Once the will is made up and the sincerity is entire, the lower nature, the external Prakriti, drops away by itself and the enlightened higher Nature takes its place.

Prakriti has to be replaced by Shakti. Lower nature has to yield to divine Nature. That is the course of sadhana in Integral Yoga. The field of nature is not to be rejected. With the shift upwards from Prakriti to Shakti, the whole direction of the life movement automatically changes. And each individual realisation has a dynamic effect on those around. Each successive victory of a soul over its lower, external nature, has a simultaneous and parallel effect on fellow sadhaks. It contributes to the strength of the soul in others on an occult level. That is what Sri Aurobindo means when he says that in a collective sadhana the victory of each sadhak has a great positive effect on the sadhana of others. So whether others are progressing and doing their part individually and collectively or not, the ideal seeker minds his own achievements, because it is truly the best help he can render to others.

How to get rid of the ego?

The ego is not something that will easily be eliminated; it survives in a hundred forms. There are many " avatars ", incarnations, of the ego. There is the physical ego, the vital ego of the life-force, the mental ego, and the highest and the worst form, the spiritual ego. This latter one feels: "I am spiritual, I am superior to all others. I am helping them; pity flows from me." This is the worst form of ego because for a man who claims to be spiritual—who perhaps has a certain spiritual nature in some part of his being—it is least excusable to have such an ego.

The ego-point is ultimately a fiction; it has no real truth. It eventually yields and merges into the truth of which it is a simulacrum. When it merges, it has fulfilled itself. In our language we may say that the ego is dead, but actually in the course of evolution, seen in the proper context, it has served its purpose of centralisation. And once the true being has emerged, the ego merges with it. Though the analogy may not completely hold good, in divine love the lover and the beloved as two entities

last only up to a certain stage; when the divine beloved
reveals itself, the lover just merges. There is none thereafter to love or waiting to be loved. There is only one
reality—that is fulfilment, it is not the death of love;
it is a crown of love. Each formation by nature has a
purpose. Once the purpose is fulfilled its part is over.
It has not been useless, but to prolong its existence after
its use is over is a perversity of which only man is
capable.

*Is it true that falsehood is dying or dead in the inner realms
of existence?*

Yes, that is true. Falsehood has been rooted out
from its base in evolution. Falsehood is a product of the
original inconscience, nescience, emerging as ignorance.
This ignorance and its product, separativity—separation of each from all others, separation of the universe
from the creator—developed into the formation called
falsehood, the very antithesis of truth. But now, with the
emergence of the supramental truth in principle, falsehood has no rightful existence. As long as truth had not
revealed itself in a plenary fashion on Earth, falsehood
could survive. But with the advent of the supramental
truth on Earth, the age of truth has begun. The era of
falsehood is fading. So whoever puts his weight on the
side of truth finds his task easier then it ever was before.
The pull of inconscience and falsehood is not so strong
on the seeker today as it was, say, even a decade ego.

We have seen how the downward pull and the
obsessive difficulties of the nether nature have lost their
power and the terror that they once held. We have only
to aspire intensely in order for the help to come and the
difficulties to lose their edge. If difficulties survive persistently, it is because something in our nature still

clings to them. If we are sufficiently sincere in our self-introspection, we can spot the erring member.

How do we free ourselves from falsehood?

We have to turn it over to the Divine to whom we have dedicated ourselves and, as a follow-up action, never listen to falsehood's suggestions. In this we must be firm, and make it a habit to offer any falsity to the Divine. As Mother once told me: give falsehood a knock on its nose every time it raises its face.

After all, it is not our own strength that can deal with such problems. If we are open, we are carried by a great and conscious power of truth. We have only to tune ourselves to it, to invoke it to act, and it deals with the situation. But as long as we have the separative sense of the doer—"I am the sadhak, and I alone fight the battle"—there is difficulty. Once we surrender ourselves centrally, it is then a process of working out the surrender in detail; surrender in detail: that is the heart of the sadhana.

What is the difference between the superman and the supramental being?

The superman is not a supramental being. The superman is the next evolutionary species after the human stage is transcended. His human mind develops in principle into its original prototype, the supermind. He is in possession of the truth at that level. That truth and its self-effectuating will are at the summit of his being. But the whole of his being is not yet transformed in terms of the consciousness of the supramental.

When the whole being, down to the material cells, is transformed in terms of the supramental conscious-ness, when the force of disintegration, death, and mortality are completely conquered and the entire system is a real physical embodiment of the divine consciousness without deviation, diminution, or dilution, that is the supramental being. That supramental being can manifest on Earth only after a race of supermen have organised life for that purpose. The superman is what the Mother and Sri Aurobindo call the intermediate race between man and the supramental being.

And Sri Aurobindo has sufficiently distinguished the superman of his conception from the superman of the German philosopher, Nietzche. It is a higher being than man, in possession of the truth-mind, the supreme light, but not yet completely transformed. Until that principle of the supramental truth has fully organised and effectuated itself in the body of Earth and negated the forces of mortality, the supramental consciousness cannot be said to have been completely manifested on Earth. First, the descent of the supramental principle has to take place, just as the descent of the mind took place aeons ago. And as it took millions of years for man, the mental being, to become the established lord of creation, there will be a time gap between the first touch of the supramental consciousness, force, and power on Earth and its gradual extension, organisation, and full establishment. So the descent, one may say, is the inception of an eventual manifestation of the supramental consciousness.

At what point of manifestation has this new consciousness arrived?

The organisation of the supramental consciousness has arrived at an articulate stage. When we speak of the consciousness of the superman, it means the Earth evolution in a certain centre of manifestation has come to a stage where that consciousness can be articulated in the form of a superman. Before this it was just a possibility, a light that had broken through and taken root on Earth. After its appearance, it has to spread, grow, and embody itself in an appropriate form, the superman. And there is a still larger step to be covered before the supramental being can emerge. But at present, anyone who opens to that universality of consciousness and divine love and who exceeds the ego can become a superman.

This possibility was not present fifteen years ago or even on the 29th of February 1956 when the descent of the supramental light took place and opened the gates as it were. Whatever has continued to pour out thereafter has to be channelised, shaped, and given a certain personality so to ultimately express itself as a superman.

The mental consciousness, for instance, is extended over the whole of creation. Even animals have a certain mind. But it is only at the human stage that mind comes into a definite, self-conscious stage. Similarly, we can say, the supramental consciousness has arrived at a self-conscious, self-effective, self-aware stage on Earth. But the road to transformation is still to be trodden, is being trodden.

It is said that the evolution will be quicker now. How is that so?

It is because it is not nature in ignorance that is now evolving; it is illumined Nature, divine Nature, that is at work. And awakened men are opening and allowing themselves to function as channels of the higher Nature, the manifesting Godhead. They are fully awakened beings. And that makes all the difference. As Sri Aurobindo says, the whole evolution from man to God can be compressed in a single lifetime provided there is the will and necessary drive. Left to nature, it would take thousands of years; but now it can be done in fifty or a hundred years. Similarly, now that the supramental force is on Earth, things will be telescoped in an unimaginable manner. What has gone on before was a solid, slow preparation for the stage of precipitation that is now at hand. The past can give no comparison to what is to happen now.

What is the role of the Matrimandir in relation to the supramental consciousness?

It is both an instrument and an expression of it. The Matrimandir is an instrument for manifesting the consciousness to which it is to be a living monument. Also, as the consciousness forms itself in the mould of the supramental truth, the Matrimandir will be its material expression. The more it rises, the wider and firmer a base it gives to the supramental in the physical matter of Earth. The Mother wants this consciousness to be received and made living not only in the human body but in all matter. The success of the Matrimandir will be, in a sense, the measure, the barometer, of the success of the manifestation of the supramental consciousness, the consciousness for transformation, on Earth.

14

EQUALITY AND THE ANNIHILATION OF EGO

Before we address ourselves to the subject of our study today, I have an important announcement to make on the Mother's behalf.

If on occasion Mother acts on her own without waiting for human conditions to be ready, there are instances when she acts only in response to the human call. An event that took place two days ago brought home to me this truth of her working.

A young, intelligent, and percipient visitor wrote to the Mother that he had been captured by the idea and spirit of Auroville. But he had a question. Are not the old forms of greeting like the folding of palms, *namaste,* or the handshake out of place in a new creation in the making like Auroville? Would it not be fitting that Aurovilians have their own, distinct mode of salutation? When he gave the letter to me, I was not inclined to take it seriously, but something in me was aware of a deeper import. So I took it up to Mother. And, true enough, she did not treat it in a light manner. She first went into meditation and afterward, with a gentle half-smile, observed that many things were coming. But she did not say anything. I asked without respite what, for instance, was coming. She took a piece of paper and on it wrote:

30.10.1972
Au service de la Verite
At the service of Truth
Truth

Thus she has given a dynamic content to the form of salutation.

In uttering any of these three alternatives, I first affirm my dedication to Truth. And this constant affirmation leads to a confirmation of the consecration in my consciousness. Further, it reminds the one I greet of this basis of Truth on which we meet. Truth is the base, Truth is the relation, Truth is the ideal towards which we both strive. With this understanding, there is no room for any of the old movements of ignorance, falsehood, and egoism to vitiate the contact any more.

Each meeting becomes an occasion for my aspiration for Truth to articulate itself, and to awaken that aspiration wherever it is dormant by the power of the conscious word.

Truth in thought, Truth in speech, towards Truth we move.

I have the privilege of communicating this message to all of you here and, through you, to all who are staying in Auroville.

And secondly, though it is not a message and though I have not been asked to communicate it, there is a recent prayer from Mother that I feel I should share with you. I have made it a point to note anything that takes place when I go to Mother that has some relevance to your endeavour here of building a new consciousness.

Most of us are hardly aware of our real defects. As one grows, however, life-experience teaches one, through a series of shocks and disillusionments, something of the truth of oneself. One begins to admit to oneself those weaknesses which are too glaring to escape notice. But that is only the first step, a new straight view which reveals something of one's nature. It is really when one turns to spiritual life and develops sincerity that one comes to realise the existence of more—in fact much more— serious defects, defects that one would not like to admit to others. All the same, it is a measure of progress that one becomes conscious of the full extent of one's failings, the nature of one's recalcitrant parts, the hold of the unspiritual elements on one's being. That, too, is not the end. As one develops in the inner consciousness, and imbibes more and more of its purity, sincerity and truth, this awareness of one's radical defects—especially when they are unspiritual or anti-divine—becomes galling. There is a sense of helpless defeat on such occasions. However, if one remembers Sri Aurobindo's injunction that one should not make too much of one's defects, then one can look forward. One can appeal to the Mother in silent prayer and she sees one through.

All this came to my mind vividly this morning when I had to talk to the Mother about a friend in similar difficulties. This friend has always impressed me with something noble in her being, with a certain dignity with which she bears some unmistakable suffering. She is gifted in many ways and, I would say, the richest gift of God that she has is sincerity. That is why she has always been conscious of a strong trait in her personality which, she says, is sadistic, perverse, hostile to what is divine or what leads to the Divine. This awareness acquired a deep poignancy after she came to the Ashram. She has undergone untold psychological suffering at every remembrance of this evil in her, and a consuming struggle ensued. She did not know whether it was right for her to stay her in this atmosphere of love, beauty, and harmony built by the Mother. As it often happens in such crises, dark thoughts of all kinds, especially self-condemnatory, overwhelmed her. Fortunately, she wrote

the Mother a frank and soulful letter expressing her
state of mind, her own evaluation of her deficiencies and
hostilities, mental and vital, and prayed to the Mother
to help her get rid of this " devil " in her. "What should
I do?" she asked.

When I put this matter before Mother, she was
moved. She went into a trance and, when she came out
of it, asked if my friend could pray. I said yes. Then she
said, "When these attacks come, let her pray to the
Divine to make her worthy of Him." She added, with
emphasis, "I have done something. I shall write a prayer
for her." She wrote in French:

27.10.1972
Seigneur de bonte, rends moi digne de Ta Grace.
And then in English:

27.10.1972
Lord of Mercy, make me worthy of Thy Grace.

That very afternoon, when the person met me, she
was completely relaxed and smiling. With tears in her
eyes, she asked if I had spoken to Mother that day. I
said that I had. She asked me at what time. When I
told her, she said that at precisely that time she suddenly felt a warm glow around her face, an unusual rush
of love, and had become very much at ease.

This prayer is for everyone of us who has evolved
enough to be conscious of his radical defects and has the
courage to admit them and the sincerity to want to get
rid of them.

We have come to a point in our study of the yoga
of works where we have agreed that the only way to
submit ourselves to the supreme will, to let our human
consciousness be taken up in the divine consciousness,

is through a complete self-consecration. This entire and detailed consecration proceeds through three well-defined stages. First comes the decision and the will to consecrate ourselves; whether or not we immediately succeed in translating this will into practice is another matter. But when we start our work, when we pause during it, and when we end it, we must affirm our will for consecration. By this constant affirmation of the will, we develop a need in our nature to consecrate. Then, though we may work, we will not have the joy, happiness, and satisfaction of the work unless it is consecrated. So this feeling of the need of consecration is the second stage. The third is when consecration develops into a natural habit. One does not have to exert one's will any longer or be reminded by a felt need in the being. One spontaneously consecrates all that one does. This is the first movement towards surrender.

The second movement is the development of a complete equality towards work. And how does this sense of equality grow? First, when one works one should give up the desire for the fruit of work. Naturally, when work is done the fruit is bound to come. But whether it corresponds to what one expects or not, the fruit should be left to the will of him to whom one consecrates the work. The Gita has declared that one has a right to action but not to the fruit of action. One offers one's labour and the fruit of that labour to the Divine. One is equal toward whatever fruit derives. This spirit of equality is cultivated first regarding the fruit of the work and then regarding the work itself. Most of us have the habit of developing attachment to the particular work we do. Whether it is due to inertia that we do not like to change our work or due to some vital satisfaction that we get from it, the fact remains that we become

attached to the work we are doing. Perhaps the work was
not even one's own choice in the beginning, but after-
wards there is still a resistance in the nature to change it.
This attachment and preference in work has to be given
up. So, we must give up the fruit of work, and also our
attachment to the work itself. Third, the sense of the
doer—"I am the worker", and even "I am the instrument"—must go. It is in the ego-centre that this
feeling persists. It takes pride in the fact that it is the
chosen instrument. This ego-point has to be dissolved.
One must realise that the real worker is the power of
God. It is a universal power, individualised so to work
through a million instruments. And each of us is but
one of these humble, limited instruments. A sense of
humility, an awareness of our own imperfections and
limitations, and a gratitude to the Divine for choosing
us as one of his instruments, have to become living to us
before the sense of equality can be established.

As in consecration, so too in the process of establishing equality there are three well-recognised stages.
First is the stage of resignation, endurance, of stoically
facing whatever comes—blows and disappointments or
successes and rejoicings. Whether experiences are good
or bad, happy or unhappy, the being presents a stoic
response. If this poise develops in the right spirit, it turns
into a submission to the will of God. The interim stage
is when one learns to withdraw from the events and
happenings of nature and take one's poise in the witness
consciousness that regards all that passes with an eye of
indifference. Sri Aurobindo calls it the philosophical
stage; the individual is not really affected by what
passes, but simply watches from above. The third stage
is when, through this separation from nature as a result
of constantly being poised nearer the uninvolved Self,

one opens to the peace and joy of the Spirit, to the divine will and knowledge and love. One feels exhilarated. The simple fact of living gives one a sense of participation in the Divine's bliss of existence. This is the culmination of the movement of equality. Whatever the occurrence or the appearance, the being remains in that peace, touches that divine bliss.

Naturally, if this sense of equality is to become really established, one must learn to recognise that it is the one Divine, the single Spirit, that is manifest in each thing in the universe. One no longer shrinks from, avoids or rejects anything in life because it is not pleasing or does not answer to one's preferences or needs. Instead of feeling repulsion or rejection, one develops a sense of understanding. One recognises that even in the ugly and cruel some divine value or power is trying to manifest. Mother said once that in the creation of God everything has its place and relevance. One recognises with sympathy, charity, and understanding that persons are what they are because of their particular stage of development and the requirements of their evolving nature. This understanding, based upon the perception of the equal pervasion of God everywhere, gives a certain release from individual reactions. And the presence of God is not merely in forms and creatures, it is also in events. Events too may be unpleasant or disappointing, but each occurrence has its meaning; each event is a result of the past and somehow a contribution to the future. The spiritual attitude in this regard is to develop an understanding and a conviction within that nothing is to be repelled, everything is to be helped to take its proper shape. There is a struggle going on everywhere in the different forms and on the different levels of life. It is the concern of the enlightened man to lend whatever helpful thoughts, emotions, and assistance he can to the establishment of harmony.

And when he sees nature in a confused or disharmonious state—whether in himself or in others—he knows that it is because of the imbalance and imperfection of the three modes of nature. These modes are: inertia and darkness; dynamism and life movement; light and peace. Till the three modes of nature attain a certain harmony and are transformed into their divine counterparts, till the lower nature is transmuted into higher Nature, friction, disharmony, and suffering are inevitable. What exactly these three modes of nature are, why they function in the way they do, and in what way they are perverted counterparts of divine values, divine modes of higher Nature, will be our next theme.

Are there any questions?

Why does Mother say to pray to Sri Aurobindo?

Mother has, I have observed, a very delicate sense of propriety and she simply would not say, " Pray to me." It is the same whether one prays to the Mother or Sri Aurobindo. It is the experience of innumerable people that theirs is a single consciousness. Both Sri Aurobindo and Mother have written to the effect that it does not matter to which of them you pray, it evokes the relevant response. And supposing someone finds it difficult to pray even to Sri Aurobindo, Mother tells them, "Pray to the Divine." Of course for us it comes to the same thing, because Sri Aurobindo and the Mother are what they are to us not as human individuals but as embodiments of the Divine. For those who have come to them as disciples or devotees, they embody the Divine. This does not mean that these two forms exhaust the Divine for the whole universe. For those who seek the Divine through them, they embody the Divine.

In the days when Sri Aurobindo was attending to correspondence, we used to address our letters to Mother, but they would be opened and answered by Sri Aurobindo. After he answered each letter or question, Mother would read his reply, write the address of the person, and send it to him. It was a way of expressing their joint working.

Does the Mother deal with people in an impersonal or a personal way?

Sri Aurobindo explained that when Mother functions from her universal aspect, she does things in an impersonal way; but when she acts from her individual aspect, she does things in a very personal way. Sri Aurobindo also, when he was dealing directly with people, used to do things in a very personal way.

A developed yogi has both these ways of functioning. At a certain level he only acts impersonally; he sends waves of peace, bliss, or dynamism. But on a frontal level he takes note of details, moulds and helps individuals and events, functions as a guru. Because the Divine has both aspects, personal and impersonal, and because, after all, man is a self-formulation of the Divine, man also has both aspects. As one develops in yoga, one can switch from the personal level to the impersonal. In the impersonal poise there is a sense of liberation and the feeling of embracing the whole universe. Though one has to cultivate both aspects, most of us have primarily to develop the impersonal poise because we are normally lost in the personal realm. Unless that impersonal status is realised, there cannot be liberation.

Even the yoga of works which is so individual in nature becomes perfect on its higher level only when it touches the impersonal realms of equality, peace, and self-surrender, only when individuality is lost and the ego is exterminated. It is in functioning from that level that one becomes more effective. Even in one's day to day work one sees—looking back over the work and into one's state at the time—it is when there is a certain impersonal consciousness or reflection of it that the work has been self-effective and automatically right. There is the swing of the right moment; all that is needed is present. That is a time when the impersonal arrangement in the occult realm concretises itself on Earth, for however brief a period.

There has been a collective experience here in the Matrimandir workers camp of a dark power attacking people at night. What is our defense? Is there some protection?

Yes. One sure method is to invoke the presence of the Mother and Sri Aurobindo before one goes to sleep and entrust oneself to them, place oneself in their hands. Meditate quietly with trust, and slide into sleep in that poise. If you do this, you will see that at the first approach of something unpleasant you will call Mother and the whole thing will dissolve. For example, in a dream it may appear as if thieves are coming to rob you. When thieves come, it means some nether forces are trying to rob you of what you have earned by your sadhana. Or it may be that some ferocious and dark beings appear. But in either case, with the repetition of the word "Mother", you can be certain that they will go. And that habit of thinking of Mother or calling her at the first unhappy reaction or occurrence has to be active in the daytime also. If one is in that poise, or goes to sleep in that poise, her consciousness and protection are

present. For one who is unable to do this, she will give—
if her attention is drawn to the need—some physical
token of her presence (a blessings packet or some
physically concentrated item) which she asks to be kept
on one's person, or under one's pillow at night. Which-
ever way it is done, one has only to call her.

It is possible that some individuals here may have
unconsciously either invited or opened themselves to
these visitations. And in a close-knit community like
this, and with the purpose it has for being, it is very
possible that the dark forces may have tried to enter. If
Mother is informed it will not continue.

*Is it possible that Matrimandir has some special attrac-
tion for these dark forces?*

Naturally. Wherever the light is to manifest and
the new is to come, the old hostile elements are bound
to try to interfere. But the opening to them will always
come through some individuals.

Why do they come particularly at night?

The balance of forces is different at night. At night
there is a preponderance of these dark elements. They
are more present at night than during the day. That is
why during the day one does not encounter these things
as much. Sri Aurobindo has described, in his *Essays on
the Gita,* how even physical light has the effect of causing
these hostile entities to recede. At night they try to gain
domination. And because man's vitality is low at night
they try to take the advantage. Particularly between
11 P.M. and 3 A.M. these forces and entities have something of a field day. But if one invokes the divine presence,
they can have no effect.

15

THE THREE MODES OF NATURE

In our study of the yoga of works we have arrived at the definitive conclusion that the lower nature which normally governs our life has to be surrendered to the Master of our being so that it may be gradually transmuted into the higher Nature which is the self-projection of the Lord. In the world, a perfectly harmonious relation with one's nature is said to be the ideal condition for successful work. But our aim is not to adjust ourselves to nature as it is, it is to exceed our nature as it is formed in ignorance and lay it before the Divine so that its character may be changed from the human to the divine nature. Before we are able to do this we must have a precise idea of what the nature is constituted.

Indian thinkers and seers have, after long observation and experiment, categorised three aspects or functionings of this nature. There is, first, the element which is called in Indian parlance, *tamas*, the principle of inertia and immobility, which translates itself into the qualities of darkness, obscurity, and ignorance. There is, next, *rajas,* the principle of kinesis, dynamism, and movement, which translates itself into the qualities of passion, force, and adventure. There is, third, *sattva,* the principle of equilibrium, which translates itself into the qualities of light, peace, and enlightenment. These three constituting qualities of nature are present wherever there is creation, individual or universal.

It is in our reaction to the impact of external nature that we can discern which part of our nature is active and dominant. If to outside impacts one's reaction is

that of acquiescence, unresisting acceptance, or uncom-
plaining sufference, it means that it is the tamas quality
that is active. If one reacts forcefully with the will to
seize contacts and utilise them, to make them an occasion to impose one's will on the environment, it is
the rajas quality that is active. If impacts are received
with a conscious, enlightened equality, assimilated as
best as possible, and responded to with waves of understanding and light, then it is the quality of sattva that is
active. No one is entirely of one nature-type. All three
are present in every individual. According to the pre-
dominant quality in his nature, a man is said to be
sattvic, rajasic, or tamasic.

When one starts yoga, the first step in dealing with
nature is to detach oneself from its movement and
observe one's nature. Through this observation you can
see of what quality your nature is in the main constituted. Nature is dynamic, and whatever the character
with which you start, in yoga you accept the possibility
of changing that nature, of transcending that nature.
If your dominant quality is that of immobility, inertia,
the refusal to enlarge and the tendency to stay put, the
obvious way to correct this rule of tamas is to awaken
the rajasic element, to invite the movements of dynamism and to evoke the forces of aspiration. If, on the
other hand, your nature is full of turbulence, restless-
ness, and the desire to dominate others and to aggran-
dise yourself, the obvious need is to stimulate the sattvic
element of understanding, enlightenment, peace, and
equilibrium, so that the turbulent elements are calmed
and controlled.

In this process of correcting the dominance of one
of the gunas by the invocation of another, it should be

remembered that no one quality always rules. If, for instance, as a yogic discipline to quiet a restless vital or control a meandering mind, you impose a stillness, there is always a tendency with the subsidence of rajas for tamas to rise and assert itself from below. With the stillness that is trying to be established or worked out, there is a strong tendency for inertia to creep in. Where rajas is suppressed, tamas comes up. Similarly, if in your desire to get out of the ignorant and obscure movements of tamas you activate the dynamic part in you and put yourself entirely in its hands, there is always the possibility of finding yourself driven by desire, rushing about in ignorance. In such a situation it is the sattvic element that has to be brought in to enlighten the rajasic. So there must, of necessity, always be a combination effected, according to the needs of the situation, between the elements of one's threefold nature.

And through observation one discovers that all three of these qualities of nature centre themselves around the ego. That is why Sri Aurobindo points out that the ego functions at different levels with different aspects, roles, and guises. There is, first, what is called the tamasic ego—the ego that cherishes its obscurity. In the very inability of the nature to move and progress, there is some part which gains a certain satisfaction. It prides itself on the fact that something is inert and will not accept any call to progress; it is satisfied that it is stable. This attachment to stability, the refusal to move, the tendency to entertain darkness especially in the form of depression, are the primary characteristics of the tamasic ego.

One of the first impediments in the way of the seeker when he takes up a yoga which calls for the change of nature is this challenge of depression. For whatever reason, for no reason at times, one experiences mental depression. It may be due to some external cause or perhaps an inner disappointment. But whatever the cause or absence of a cause, left to itself, depression passes. But the tamasic ego is attached to depression and seeks to retain it. Though it is rather difficult to believe, it is a fact that something in the tamasic nature inwardly delights in depression and suffering, and refuses to take steps to dissipate the depression. The main obstacle in the early stages of sadhana is this dominance of the tamasic ego.

Second, there is the rajasic ego, the ego of the vital which wants to assert itself and dominate whatever it can of its environment. It is not satisfied unless it extends its rule. This desire for aggrandisement may function in the domain of the mind through the imposition of ideas, on the life plane through the exercise of power to control, or even in the physical realm through physical possessiveness. The rajasic ego, unlike the tamasic ego, is very easy to recognise—especially when it is in others.

There is a third ego which is very subtle—the sattvic ego. A man who cultivates the mind, who has a certain sense of poise and equality, who can feel the light of knowledge, however distant, develops the ego of the sattvic mind if he takes an inordinate pride in his achievements and clings to the particular formulation of knowledge that he has acquired. He feels and proclaims that his knowledge is the truth, yours is not. Some are more clever, they don't proclaim it loudly but they are convinced that their ideas are the truth. They become prisoners of their ideas, prisoners of their half-knowledge. They do not progress. It is easy enough for Nature to give a kick to the tamasic ego or a shock to

the rajasic ego and make them progress. But it is
extremely difficult for a man with a sattvic ego, the ego
of knowledge, to progress. Very often, philosophers and
those who speculate and weave systems of thought
refuse to look beyond their walls, they close the windows
of their minds, and they become possessed of this sattvic
ego.

And then, there is what is called the spiritual ego.
When a man touches even the fringe of the higher consciousness or receives in himself some ingression of the
higher being, influence, or force, he has the tendency
to feel that he has arrived and is superior to others. He
feels kindly towards others and he likes to feel kindly.
He feels that those around him are unfortunate people
who need his help and that it is incumbent upon him
to go to them, to lead them, to make them his disciples
and give them the benefit of his guidance. This pride of
piety, as it is called, this egoism of spirituality, is the
worst form of ego. It is the worst because it is all the
more inexcusable for one who claims to be open to light
and in possession of a higher consciousness to allow the
play of ego even at that stage.

For one who is still in the belt of ignorance and
darkness and obscurity, ego is perhaps natural. But it is
absolutely impermissible and unnatural in a spiritual
seeker who has imbibed even something of the spiritual
consciousness.

The three qualities of nature in the being, organised
around the ego at different levels, have to be transcended. And transcended they can be, because these
formations of all three qualities are not the real, original
forms of their higher principles. Just as matter, life, soul,
and mind are inverted projections of existence, consciousness-force, bliss, and supermind, similarly the

three gunas of sattva, rajas, and tamas are projections
of three higher spiritual qualities which in their involution into ignorance have taken these forms. What is
called tamas, the principle of inertia and immobility, is
really a deformation of that which is on the heights of
the being tranquility and immutable stability. What is
called rajas, the principle of kinesis, is a projection of the
consciousness-force radiating the power and light of the
truth behind. And what is called sattva, the principle
of equilibrium, is derived from the light, undisturbed
peace, and quiet certainty of truth-knowledge. The three
lower formations of the gunas are gradually transmuted
into their divine, higher equivalents as they are surrendered to the Master of our being and his puissance,
the Shakti.

Incidentally, this perversion of the three qualities
of sattva, rajas, and tamas is described in the seven-
teenth chapter of the Gita as far as it pertains to our
food, to sacrifice, and to our sadhana. When the Gita
speaks of sacrifice, it does not so much mean the physical
act of sacrifice as it does the inner act of adoration and
worship. It says:

"Sattwic men offer sacrifice to the gods, the rajasic
to the Yakshas (the keepers of wealth) and the Raksha-
sic forces; the others, the tamasic, offer their sacrifice to
elemental powers and grosser spirits. [These are the
supernatural entities on the lower level of the higher
hemisphere.]

"The men who perform violent austerities, contrary to the Shastra, with arrogance and egoism,
impelled by the force of their desires and passions, men
of unripe minds tormenting the aggregated elements
forming the body and troubling Me also, seated in the

body, know these to be Asuric in their resolves. [Asuric means perverted Rajasic.]

"The food also which is dear to each is of triple character, as also sacrifice, askesis and giving. Hear thou the distinction of these.

"The sattwic temperament in the mental and physical body turns naturally to the things that increase the life, increase the inner and outer strength, nourish at once the mental, vital and physical force and increase the pleasure and satisfaction and happy condition of mind and life and body, all that is succulent and soft and firm and satisfying.

"The rajasic temperament prefers naturally food that is violently sour, pungent, hot, acrid, rough and strong and burning, the aliments that increase ill-health and the distempers of the mind and body.

"The tamasic temperament takes a perverse pleasure in cold, impure, stale, rotten or tasteless food or even accepts like the animals the remnants half-eaten by others.

"The sacrifice which is offered by men without desire for the personal fruit, which is executed according to the right principle, and with a mind concentrated on the idea of the thing to be done as a sacrifice, that is sattwic.

"The sacrifice offered with a view to the personal fruit, and also for ostentation, know thou that to be of a rajasic nature.

"The sacrifice not performed according to the right rule of the Shastra, without giving of food, without the mantra, without gifts, empty of faith, is said to be tamasic.

"Worship given to the godhead, to the twice-born, to the spiritual guide, to the wise, cleanness, candid dealing, sexual purity and avoidance of killing and injury to others, are called the askesis of the body.

"Speech causing no trouble to others, true, kind and beneficial, the study of Scripture, are called the askesis of speech.

"A clear and calm gladness of mind, gentleness, silence, self-control, the purifying of the whole temperament—this is called the askesis of the mind."

There is even a classification of the way of giving to others.

"The sattwic way of giving is to do it for the sake of the giving and the beneficence and to one who does no benefit in return; and it is to bestow in the right conditions of time and place and on the right recipient (who is worthy or to whom the gift can be really helpful).

"The rajasic kind of giving is that which is done with unwillingness or violence to oneself or with a personal and egoistic object or in the hope of a return of some kind.

"The tamasic gift is offered with no consideration of the right conditions of time, place and object; it is offered without regard for the feelings of the recipient and despised by him even in the acceptance."[1]

This reflects the all-pervading nature of the triple qualities of lower nature, Prakriti, as it is called in Indian terminology. One has to cultivate the higher gunas,

1. Anilbaran Roy, ed., *The Gita: With Text, Translation and Notes, Compiled from Sri Aurobindo's "Essays on the Gita"* (London: George Allen & Unwin Ltd., 1946), pp. 236-40, 242-43.

transmute each lower formation into its original one, and arrive at a higher state of detachment by the cultivation of stoic endurance, indifference, and equality. One is thus freed from the domination of the gunas through the practice of sadhana.

But the freedom from the gunas is not the final aim. It is only an indispensable basis for the transcendence of the gunas. One must rise above the gunas so to control them, to force them to change and serve as vehicles for the higher consciousness. When the three qualities of equilibrium, kinesis and stability function in terms of the higher consciousness, they are a great asset for the manifestation that is ahead.

16

THE MASTER OF THE WORK

We have been considering the way of doing works fruitfully in yoga, the process of converting works from labour into service to God and a means for our spiritual evolution. Instead of allowing work to become a means of bondage and the forge of karma, we have discussed how it can be elevated into a means of our release from ego and of identification with the Divine.

And who is the Divine to whom our works stand consecrated? Who is the Master who claims the allegiance of our personality? The Master of our works, says Sri Aurobindo, is the Supreme, none less than the Eternal, the One of whom the world and much more are the expression. He is the transcendental Absolute, beyond all the formulations that we have known and are yet to know. He is the Divine manifested in and as the universe of which each one of us is a significant part. He is also the indweller whose presence charges every living form. He takes more poises than one: the individual poise in man, the universal poise in the cosmos, and the transcendental poise beyond. It is to him that our life should stand consecrated, to him that our works must be offered in loving consecration.

But it is not easy for man as he is, shut up in his prison of lower nature and egoism, to straightaway achieve this consummation. There is a process, and the process is long. None can really establish a link with the Master unless he first renounces the egoism of the worker. The feeling that I am the worker should go. It should be replaced by the knowledge that I am only an in-

strument of the power of the Lord, only the shakti of
the Master to whom I am dedicated. It is not easy to
dislodge this ego which masquerades in various guises.
And when this egoism of the worker is eliminated, there
is still the egoism of the instrument. One develops a
pride of being the chosen channel, an instrument pre-
ferred by the Divine over others, who are for that reason
inferior. This egoism is also to be overpassed.

It is possible that the seeker on this path may be
granted a vision of the Master at the very beginning of
his adventure. It is possible that he may be visited by
illuminations, visions, and experiences testifying to the
presence of the Master and the workings of the dynamic
Shakti. But that is not a culmination. We are asked to
remember that they are only initial openings, happy and
promising no doubt, but they are not the end. To have
seen the vision, to have been given the *darshan* of the
Supreme is a boon, indeed. But it is only a beginning.
Only if one undergoes the long and strenuous labour of
digging in one's consciousness, and of building in oneself the image of the ideal, will the promise of those
initial experiences have been fulfilled.

It requires a tremendous faith and an unfailing
patience to tread this path of consecration leading to
the Master of our being. When one commences the
journey there is an initial enthusiasm, a great desire to
get away from the humdrum world and existence and
to change oneself. With this combination of rajasic
eagerness, the enthusiasm of the heart, and the restless-
ness of the mind, one seeks to storm the kingdom of
heaven and take it by force. When one fails to do so,
there is a reaction of disappointment and depression,
and the faith wavers. It is at such moments that one has
to remember that the path is long and the divine prize

is not won easily. As is said in one of the Upanishads, it is the path of the razor's edge. One must persist, and fortify the initial faith. The reason will deny what faith affirms, but we know that faith is a projection in our being of a light that is other than that of the mind. The certainty of faith is a reflection of a divine will above. Faith is wiser than our reason and more steadfast than our human will.

And because of the character of the path, one needs patience. When one begins, one is aware of only a limited part of one's nature. But as one goes deeper, more and more regions are exposed to the light and one becomes aware of the much that is not normally seen or known. Human nature is full of imperfections, but it is not given to the seeker of the integral path to reject the whole of his nature; it will not do to leave nature to itself as the ascetic or the nihilist does. One has to accept nature with all its imperfections and subject it to the pressure of transmutation and change. A rigorous discipline, sincerely followed, must be imposed on nature so that step by step, part by part, this lower human nature is changed into its higher term. Yet one must remember that man is not alone in this experiment. The Divine to whom one surrenders and opens helps. The Divine is felt in the heart of the seeker in a hundred ways.

The One is not only above, he is around, and he is within. And it is one of the objects of the Integral Yoga to realise in oneself all the three statuses of the supreme Divine. That is possible because deep within each one of us there is a spark, a ray of the Divine. In the course of evolution it develops and affirms itself as the individual Divine. When one has taken to or is driven to the path of yoga, one can be sure that one has arrived at a point in evolution where the divine personality within has started forming itself. If one can withdraw one's gaze from external preoccupations and direct it inward and can relate all movements of life and all items of work to this centre in the heart, to this presence which one should learn to feel concretely, the whole character of life begins to change. One forms a new centre of reference and it becomes the focus of one's life and energies. One lives from within. One is fully established in the status of the individual Divine.

And then there is an effortless outflow into the universe, the cosmic being: "the island ego joins its continent". The tiny bit of the Divine embodied in the individual being joins a larger being. One feels a certain effortless unity with other individualisations of the Divine. It is a sign of the spiritual development of an individual when he is able to perceive in others the same divinity which is within himself. It is not a mental formula or theory, it is a spontaneous perception, an experience which impinges upon the consciousness.

And it is this perception and experience that has given rise to the famous exaltation in the Upanishads that it is not for the love of the wife that she is dear to the husband, but for love of the Self a wife is dear. One recognises the divinity in others. This recognition flows in the form of love and attraction, though on the ignorant human level it may be tainted by ego and desire. But the truth stands that at the heart of every genuine attraction there is this mutual recognition of the same divine manifest in two individuals.

This extension of the individual realisation to the universal realisation changes the whole character of work and enlarges its range. There is no longer conflict between the work undertaken by one who has attained this realisation and the work undertaken by others. All work falls into a harmonious pattern because each element is a segment of a whole which has been pre-visioned by the truth-being above.

Above whom and above what? Above this triple formula of the cosmos. This universe does not exhaust the Divine. The universe lives by That, but That does not live by the universe. In a famous hymn of the Rig Veda it is recorded that the Divine Being made a holocaust of himself and projected the whole creation out of himself. Having done it, he exceeded the universe by nine digits; this is a metaphor reflecting the truth that he stands beyond, only a part of himself is manifested here on Earth and in the universe.

This transcendent poise of consciousness must also be realised for there to be a full perfection. A great liberation is possible through the universal realisation; but perfection of the kind envisaged for the spiritually evolving man is not possible within the existing term of the divine expression in the universe. A still higher truth has to be manifested. The mind has to leap beyond itself. The worker has to project his vision above the universal formula and, through the psychic, link himself with his transcendent origin. One has to ascend to transcendent heights, and one has also to descend with the transcendent truth. This double play of ascent and descent to and from the transcendent is the culmination of the ages-long endeavour of man to realise in himself the perfect figure of his Maker. For, beyond the highest heights of the mind there stands the gnosis—the truth-idea, the divine truth self-formulated as knowledge and as will inseparable from that knowledge—in which the universe to be manifest is made ready. It is previsioned and preconceived in seed form, in what Sri Aurobindo calls the real-idea.

Each form in the universe has behind it its own relevant real-idea. This real-idea determines the precise line of development and expression of each ray of the Infinite; it determines the way in which each form is to fulfil itself, is to express its particular stress of manifestation. And all these real-ideas form a natural whole in the supermind, in the great Real-Idea where knowledge is self-evident. Truth is self-radiating, and that knowledge's perception carries a spontaneous power to effectuate itself.

It is only when one reaches this gnostic level that the whole of human nature stands a chance of being completely transmuted into divine Nature. There is at that level a natural harmonisation of the different poises of the creative Divine—the transcendental, the universal, and the individual. That harmony and oneness is not gained by an arithmetical totalling to arrive at the One. But there is a simultaneous formation of the three aspects or poises of the one Reality. The Master of our works and being is there above us and around us, but he is also here in the heart of each one of us. Through the heart lies the path. In the mind opens the vision. The aim is to renounce the ego.

And how is the ego to be renounced? One must dedicate all work, that is, all that one does on the planes of thinking, feeling, and acting. On all three planes of work, one consecrates each action to the Divine. The test of this consecration is in the offering of the fruits of the work. Once one offers work to the Divine, the result, the fruit, is the Divine's concern. To offer oneself and to feel the Divine's presence and his acceptance

of the fruit is itself sufficient. After renunciation of the
fruit of work comes the renunciation of the sense of the
worker. And after renunciation of the egoism of the
worker comes the renunciation of the pride of the instrument. It is only once these steps have been taken
that there is a release, that the inner psychic personality
comes to the front and guides and illumines the various
activities of the being. Surrender works out the rest.
The way is opened for perfect identification with the
Divine on all the planes of our being.

I have been asked to answer a question which is of
interest because most of us have experienced, or will
likely experience at some time in our inner life, the
phenomenon it concerns.

When I have a spiritual experience or when I feel
I have overcome certain deficiencies in my being or a
long-standing illness, if I speak about it to someone, that
experience stops or that chronic illness comes back.
This happens even if I don't speak to someone but merely
say to myself, "I have achieved something", or "Now
it is over." If mentally I make such a formulation,
either in word or thought, it often happens that the
experience stops or the deficiencies or illnesses return.
That which seemed to have been achieved is lost.

Why does this happen? There are two possible
explanations. When we say to somebody else or to ourselves, "I have done this, I am now free", the hostiles—
who are always waiting for an occasion to interfere and
to strike—rush into the situation and say, as it were,
"You say so do you? We will prove to you that it is not
so." And they proceed to upset the whole poise, to
negate whatever has been experienced.

The second explanation is even less generally known. Just as there are in the creation many gods, powers, or deities presiding over their particular domains and exercising their particular functions, there are also in the individual atmosphere certain agents—called in the Vedas, the *nidas* or in occult science, the censors— who are always on the watch. They will not allow one who is serious about spiritual progress to progress beyond the vision and level to which he is accustomed, unless he fulfils the evolutionary conditions and require- ments of that stage. They will not allow one to cross into the next higher belt unless one earns that right. Till then, they will continue to suggest to you, through others or your own mind, that you have failed, that this is your defect, that you are not attending to this. They never miss an opportunity to point out your defects and defi- ciencies, and impress upon you the much that is still to be done.

This phenomenon is of great occult significance. One has to learn to discriminate because these censors also have a habit of exaggerating things. I have known many people who have fallen victim to the tricks of these censors. One can completely lose sight of the positive side of things and become preoccupied with searching for and imagining defects where there are none, in oneself and in others. This tendency has to be resisted. But a discriminate attention does have to be paid to the activities and indications of these censors.

Till an experience is wholly confirmed, fully orga- nised, and firmly established in the being, Mother says the best thing is not to formulate it in words or in thought but to allow it to grow without thinking or talking about it. There are even instances where speaking of an experience to one's teacher can cause it to stop. But of course there are teachers of different types; one has to discriminate. Ordinary human gurus of the type that abound in the world are not always happy at the too rapid progress of their disciples. Naturally, with a divine teacher like the one that we are fortunate to have, this won't happen. Divine or divinely appointed teachers always put a fresh impulsion for the experience to grow. When an experience matures into a realisation it can stand any amount of formulation or verbal expression. Till then it is not safe to discuss it in one's own mind or with others.

If one makes this error of thinking or talking about an experience prematurely, how can one recoup what is lost?

In God's scheme of things, such gains are never entirely lost. When an experience has taken place it does leave some concrete impression on the being. The experience can be re-evoked and re-established. And having learnt this lesson, the experience can become even stronger. No spiritual experience is ever completely lost. Even when a person dies before an experience can be completed, it is taken up in the next incarnation from the precise point where it stopped.

Some speak of their experiences in order to help others. What happens in this case?

Some are so self-giving that they simply don't mind the risk. But it is also always possible to give the benefit of an experience to others without bringing in the personal element. One does not need to say, "I have had this experience." And if one's experience is genuine, the moment one speaks of it, something of that experience is communicated to those who are open. But it is only a living experience that can make a living impact. If the experience is sufficiently confirmed, certainly one can speak about it if that will help another. But if one has a concealed desire to parade one's superiority and to impress others with one's experience—there is the danger. If it is just to show that one is advanced and has gone further than others, what one says ultimately falls flat anyway.

For the manifestation of the divine truth, is not something more needed than just an understanding of what is to be expressed?

Yes, there is another element necessary. Even though one may have the mental knowledge, the perception, or even the spiritual vision of the truth that is to be manifested and organised, below the supramental level, the full will power and dynamism that can translate that knowledge into a reality is not present. That full power is active only on the plane of the truth-being, the gnosis, the supramental. Here there is always a lacuna between knowledge and will. If there is the will, the knowledge of what to do is lacking. If there is the knowledge, the will for it to be effectuated is lacking. It is only on the truth plane that knowledge and will are coexistent. They are two sides of the same reality.

When knowledge and will are one, is then the full divine manifestation in the individual you spoke of possible?

Such a plenary manifestation of the Divine will be possible only when the supramental consciousness is fully organised on Earth and can work in the individual without the obstacles of his lower nature arising. Of course no complete descent of the supramental consciousness or light is possible until these barriers are broken and the whole individual system is transmuted into terms of the divine Nature. Complete manifestation can take place in the individual only on the basis of the full realisation of the supermind. The beginnings of that manifestation on Earth occur only when a first individual on Earth is fully supramentalised.

Could you comment on Mother's statement of 26 November 1972, in which she spoke of the complete necessity of Truth in terms that she has not used before: "Before dying falsehood rises in full swing. Still people understand only the lesson of catastrophe. Will it have to come before they open their eyes to the truth? I ask an effort from all so that has not to be. It is only the Truth that can save us; truth in words, truth in action, truth in will, truth in feeling. It is a choice between serving the Truth or being destroyed."

This situation has been gathering for some time now. Mother has been repeatedly speaking of it. She said that there was a time when people used to be afraid to tell lies in her presence. But now, she remarked, people come to her and tell her lies with a smile. It is, in part, this phenomena that has necessitated her message. I have observed that Mother tolerates any weakness, forgives anything, but she abhors falsehood. She cannot countenance a lie.

The present time is certainly one where Truth is acting with full pressure on the existing falsehood—in the general atmosphere, in individuals, and in the collectivity. Falsehood is making its last effort to express itself and to resist the incoming Truth. In a certain sense, it ultimately depends on each one of us which way things will go. The divine will is acting for the victory of Truth. But it will not precipitate unprepared—for conditions on Earth—as Sri Aurobindo noted in the chapter we have just now discussed. The Divine respects our nature even as he works upon it. The Earth, the Earth-consciousness, and the sadhaks and seekers who have gathered here and elsewhere, still have the freedom to choose between Truth and falsehood. If by their thoughts and actions they put their weight on the side of falsehood, the Truth will recede and wait for another occasion. This is one implication of Mother's words. The only reason the Truth would have to recede is if falsehood continues to be harboured by those who are gathered here in quest of the supramental ideal. The way Mother has put it underlies that it is an individual choice between Truth and falsehood which is posing itself.

17

THE DIVINE WORK AND THE SUPERMIND

In our discussion so far we have traced the development of the seeker in the way of works to the point where he has become a perfect vehicle for the Divine. We have analysed the various elements of the path, the way in which it is to be tread, the difficulties and dangers that face the seeker, and the consummation at which he arrives by his own effort seconded by divine grace.

By this stage, the seeker has eliminated from himself not only the last traces of ego, but also of egoity. He has taken care to shed the shadows of egoism not merely from the dynamic parts of his outer nature, but also from his psychological being. He has eliminated personal desire in both the choice of work and in the preference for fruits. He has patiently worked out the successive steps of his consecration and translated his central determination to surrender to the Divine in terms of his daily life; in each step of his work, in every expenditure of his energy, he has taken care to cultivate the attitude of self-consecration. From being a worker he has developed into an instrument; from being an instrument he has grown into a channel of the divine presence; from the experience of the mere presence of the Divine, he has moved into contact with the Lord of works, the Master of his being. Having arrived at this stage, what more remains for the worker? Must he still do work or is he expected to withdraw into the bliss of the Self, into the silence that breathes of the transcendent?

There are traditions, notably in India, which enjoin this course of withdrawal. They look upon work as part of an inferior movement. For them, work must be done, indeed, but as part of the life of ignorance which is imposed upon the developing soul. It is, therefore, necessary only as long as one is within the belt of ignorance. If by some means one has risen above that realm, the doing of works is no longer binding. Not only are works not a binding requirement, but they are considered a nuisance and a standing danger that may cause one to slip back into the bonds of karma. Some have, however, condescended to look upon work as a means for working out one's karma and, as a concession to the ordinary man, to not disturb the faith of those who are still in ignorance. This entire attitude toward work is erroneous.

Then there are those who say that the seeker who has arrived at this consummation has no obligation to work for himself but that he has a duty to society. It is perfectly right that a spiritual man must render service to humanity, to the world, but on the condition that it is the Master of works in humanity he regards and serves. Even if one has realised God in one's sadhana and daily life, it is incomplete unless it is extended into the realisation of the universal Godhead. And the Godhead in the universe does not exist in a vacuum. He exists in everything around us. The Divine is everywhere. The service that an enlightened seeker has to render is to God in the world and society, at all levels of creation.

If one has this conception, is alive to this truth, then service to humanity has a meaning. Individually, one has no claim and does not choose what work is to be done. None of the human standards which have been erected for the ordinarily evolving soul are applicable to him. Indian wisdom has long recognised this freedom for the liberated soul. It has given him an utter freedom to do what he chooses, what he is moved to do. Though indeed this freedom has on occasion been misused, that is no reason why one should not see the truth of the liberty given to the genuine seeker. Each movement of thought and action from a liberated man proceeds from a source other than the human. For he has contacted and is in union with the individual Divine stationed at the core of his being. His external consciousness is in tune with, is on the right wavelength to catch the vibration of, the intention of the Lord seated within. He does not care whether the action that he does conforms to the social and other standards reigning at the moment. All that he is concerned with is receiving the command and carrying it out.

A seeker who has arrived at this stage of realisation may outwardly appear not very different from others or he may be a world-shaking figure. He may choose to abide by all the rules and standards that govern the society in which he lives or he may be led to shake its very foundations, to destroy them and attempt a new creation. All depends upon the divine will.

Following the way of knowledge, one may arrive at a total freedom of the mind beyond the last reaches of ignorance and falsehood and perceive the Divine everywhere—in the universe and even beyond. And on the higher levels of one's awakened mind, one may breathe the air of the transcendent. Or one may follow the way of love, and the whole of the being and consciousness may melt in adoration of the Lord, become one in the flow upward with the Master. But both these movements, these spiritual realisations, are not complete unless one dynamises them in terms of action.

Unless the spiritual gains of the soul are rendered effectively in terms of work—work for the Divine in oneself
and for the Divine in others and in the creation—there
is no integral realisation. Humanity has trodden the
separate ways of realisation for centuries, but the time
has come when all the old gains have to fuse. All the
ancient paths are converging towards a new meeting
place where the static and the dynamic movement of
the creative Divine meet in the human individual.

The yoga of works lays down the basis, describes
the process and the goal. There is no one rule or way
governing the development of an individual seeker, and
certainly not a single line applicable to all. The mode of
working for each one changes from day to day. What
once appeared relevant may now seem silly. Everything
concerning the divine worker is to be evaluated from the
standpoint of the consciousness that is growing in him.
The development of consciousness is the first consideration, not the quantity of work that is done or even the
quality of work. The significance of work lies ultimately
in what has been effected as far as the deepening or the
heightening of the consciousness.

I know of instances where people have worked day
and night in order to complete assignments for the
Mother which would normally have taken a much
longer time; but still, when that work was passed on to
Mother, the moment she touched it she would say, "It
is merely labour." It took me a little while to understand that what she found missing was consciousness,
the spirit of consecration. It is not vast quantities of
mechanical work that appeals to the Divine, but it is
the link with the divine consciousness established through
that work that matters. This consideration of the spirit
in which work is done is of the utmost relevance to all

of us—whether in the Ashram, Auroville, or elsewhere in the world—who want to progress toward the divine consciousness.

Efficiency, technique, and skill are important indeed, but in their own place. Considered from the point of view of spiritual progress and evolution, it is the quality of consciousness poured out through physical, vital, and mental expenditures of energy that is of greatest import and that must be most attended to. One has to be vigilant to keep work always at a higher level, unmixed with the lower movements of action and reaction common in the environment. A sadhak cannot afford to be subject to the ordinary play of forces. He has to maintain his poise and remember why he is working and what the work means to him and his Maker. He must be conscious of the psychological and spiritual background of work.

And what will be the position of the divine worker when he attains to the supramental consciousness? Will he even then be required to work? Again the answer can only be an unqualified yes. For the consciousness of the supermind is the truth-consciousness, and it expresses itself equally in knowledge, love, will, and action. Activity will naturally continue, but with the difference that it will be fully illumined by truth-knowledge, it will be ensouled by divine love. The very nature of the supramental consciousness is to manifest the truth. In fact, the plane of the supermind has been constituted for the purpose of manifesting Sat-Chit-Ananda, Existence-Consciousness-Bliss. Every action at this level becomes a natural movement of the Eternal and the Infinite. The seeker not only ascends into the supramental truth, but he also becomes an instrument for the dynamic descent of its light and truth.

The seeker of the integral path does not strive to reach the supermind for his own sake, but for the sake of the Divine. His intention is to unite integrally with the divine Reality, and in his being to possess it and dynamise it in all possible ways. To seek the supermind for any other reason, for the glory of supermanhood for instance, is to wholly miss the ideal. And for a worker, it is doubly dangerous. For power comes inevitably with the supramental change, and unless he has the right consciousness, it is likely to lead him on the way to self-aggrandisement. He should always remember that yoga is for the Divine, for the manifestation of the Divine, not for his individual glorification.

There is another danger. One is apt to mistake high, supernormal states of consciousness for supramental states. One tends to forget that the supramental change is the ultimate stage, a far-off destination. Much is to be done before we can arrive at that consciousness. In a remarkable passage, Sri Aurobindo describes the intermediate steps that must be first taken. We must acquire an inner yogic consciousness to replace the ordinary awareness and movements of life; we must go still deeper and discover the psychic being, and with its help psychicise our inner and outer nature; we must then spiritualise the being by a descent of a divine light, force, and knowledge; we must break out of the walls of our ego, and enlarge ourselves till we enter into the cosmic consciousness and attain complete universalisation. Only then can the passage to the supramental consciousness open.

The way is long and it is tempting to try to bypass the stages or force the way. But that can only increase the risks and expose one to the danger of imbalance. A steady and sustained effort at integration at each successive level of attainment is needed, and no abnormality of any kind is permissible.

Also needed is a keen capacity of discrimination. All light is not the light of the Spirit or the supramental. There are many different lights. Each dimension of consciousness, vertical or horizontal, has its own light and force. But the light and force of the supramental are distinctive. They are fully above the reaches of ignorance, inconscience, and nescience. It is an unmixed, unmodified truth-consciousness that reigns in the supramental ranges. Further, it is not enough to achieve this high consciousness in its status, in its essence; it is indispensable to also draw up our dynamic parts into the light and working of that consciousness. Otherwise, a diminution in manifestation will occur.

Are there any questions?

Are the tools we use affected by our state of consciousness?

When one is conscious during work, that quality of consciousness is naturally imparted to what one is working with or upon. For instance, if each time you use a particular pen you are breathing a higher consciousness, functioning at a higher or deeper level, that pen does imbibe something of the consciousness vibrant in you at that time. This is the actual significance of things used by saints and seers. Such objects retain the vibration of the person who has used them, and they link one immediately with that consciousness.

Are catastrophes necessary in order to destroy the old world?

No additional cataclysms are necessary for the destruction of the old world; the destruction has already

taken place. The roots of the present civilisation have
been obliterated on the subtler levels of existence.
Physical catastrophes are no longer necessary. The unrest
visible all over the world—physical and psychological—
is due to the fact that the bearings of the old civilisation
are, indeed, already gone.

Because man today is a mental being, the destruction has occurred on the mental plane. All the cherished
ideas that were thought sufficient have been demolished.
Man knows that he has no adequate mental values or
standards to stand by. This demolition has taken place,
and things are ready on the subtler planes for the new to
organise itself. It is, as I see it, a part of this adjustment
between the receding past and the emerging new that
there are disturbances in physical Nature.

Mother has explained that when the new, higher
forces act upon the Earth-consciousness and the reception is insufficient and assimilation does not occur, there
are certain imbalances, and external results ensue—
like earthquakes, floods, or other disasters. But that does
not mean that every physical disaster has a spiritual
cause. Certain catastrophes are the work of the hostile
powers. But some are the result of imbalances caused by
resistance to the new conditions—not necessarily ill-will,
but the inability to adjust and harmonise.

If Mother has recently laid special stress on the
necessity of seeking the Truth and overpassing falsehood,
it is because she sees that progress in certain directions
is being obstructed because individuals persist in their
allegiance to untruth. One such individual is enough to
spread disaster. All are not vigilant; all are not always
conscious. One person in tune with falsehood, consciously or unconsciously, becomes a medium of hostile

forces and can sabotage a whole movement. It is as a warning against this possibility that the Mother has spoken of catastrophe. But I am a believer in Grace. Whatever the falsehoods and resistances, they will be swept away. As long as Mother is holding the force of the divine truth-consciousness on Earth, there cannot be any irretrievable disaster, natural or otherwise.

She asks from each individual here the contribution of giving up falsehood and choosing the truth at every moment. Unless we cultivate this habit of thinking, feeling, and acting truly, when the truth-consciousness tries to descend into us it will not find a home. That is what Sri Aurobindo means when he says: "You must keep the temple clean if you wish to install there the living Presence."

OTHER TITLES BY SRI M.P. PANDIT:

Dhyana (Meditation)	**1.95**
Dictionary of Sri Aurobindo's Yoga	**7.95**
Gems from the Gita	**3.95**
Gems from the Veda	**3.95**
Japa (Mantra Yoga)	**1.95**
Kundalini Yoga	**4.95**
Occult Lines Behind Life	**3.95**
Sadhana in Sri Aurobindo's Yoga	**3.95**
Spiritual Life: Theory & Practice	**7.95**
Yoga for the Modern Man	**4.00**
YOGA OF KNOWLEDGE	**in the press**
YOGA OF LOVE	**3.95**
YOGA OF SELF PERFECTION	**7.95**

available from your local bookseller or

LOTUS LIGHT PUBLICATIONS
P.O. BOX 2, WILMOT, WI 53192 USA
(414) 862-6968